In Clinical Practice

Taking a practical approach to clinical medicine, this series of smaller reference books is designed for the trainee physician, primary care physician, nurse practitioner and other general medical professionals to understand each topic covered. The coverage is comprehensive but concise and is designed to act as a primary reference tool for subjects across the field of medicine.

Ian Jones

Necrotising Enterocolitis in Clinical Practice

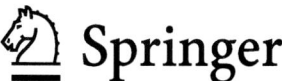 Springer

Ian Jones
Department of Paediatric Surgery
Birmingham Children's Hospital
Birmingham, UK

ISSN 2199-6652   ISSN 2199-6660   (electronic)
In Clinical Practice

ISBN 978-3-031-64147-3   ISBN 978-3-031-64148-0   (eBook)
https://doi.org/10.1007/978-3-031-64148-0

This Springer imprint is published by the registered company Springer Nature Switzerland AG
The registered company address is: Gewerbestrasse 11, 6330 Cham, Switzerland

If disposing of this product, please recycle the paper.

Preface

The arrival of a baby is a very human experience. In modern, high-income societies, infant mortality rates are a fraction of what they once were. Families look forward to the arrival of a baby with hope and optimism and joy. In most cases, premature birth is an unexpected event and the situation for the families is very different to that for which they were prepared. A baby born at a very early gestation faces many challenges. In the early part of the twenty-first century, many of these challenges are no longer insurmountable. Whilst lifelong morbidity is often a consequence of premature birth, it is not inevitable. In fact, most babies born prematurely today survive and many do so without major disability. The advancement in neonatal care of the past few decades is truly remarkable.

For a baby born too early, the first few days and weeks are challenging but with expert treatment, many progress as hoped and parents and clinical teams alike begin to become optimistic that this is a baby who will grow and develop and be discharged in good health. Then for a proportion of them NEC develops. This devastating disease changes that optimistic prognosis. The outlook for survival is no longer assured and if the baby does survive, the chance of severe life-long morbidity is now much higher.

As a paediatric surgeon, I have looked after and operated on many such babies with NEC. Most often, these are infants who follow the pattern described above, they are still very small and vulnerable but making good progress when NEC hits. It is truly tragic how NEC makes outcomes so much worse than comparable infants who—for whatever reason—did not contract NEC. As a researcher, like thousands of others, I have sought to contribute to the body of knowledge that will lead to better treatments and better outcomes.

This small volume is meant as a handy guide to the state of the art with NEC. Where we are now and where we go from here as professionals who care for the smallest babies with this horrible disease.

Birmingham, UK   Ian Jones
2024

Contents

Chapter 1
Introduction

Keywords Necrotising enterocolitis · Premature infants · Neonatal gastrointestinal disorder · Intestinal necrosis · Bowel inflammation · Infant mortality · Neonatal intensive care · Risk factors NEC · Diagnosis NEC Treatment NEC · Neonatal surgery · Gut microbiota · Enteral feeding · Antibiotic therapy · Probiotics in NEC prevention · Bell's staging criteria · Complications of NEC · Intestinal perforation · Sepsis in NEC · Long-term outcomes

Necrotising enterocolitis (NEC) is a devastating disease with both a high mortality and significant, life-long morbidity for a high proportion of survivors. Approximately nine out of ten cases occur in preterm infants but the disease is also seen in other groups of babies, primarily those born with congenital cardiac conditions. There is a broad range of clinical manifestations of the disease; in some cases babies recover completely with only conservative management. In more severe cases, babies require surgery and bowel resection. Infants with NEC can also develop systemic disease and multi-organ failure.

NEC is a rarity in medicine in that it is a genuinely modern disease that emerged as a clinical entity in the second half of the twentieth century. The majority of patients with NEC are pre-term neonates who prior to the use of incubators and the development of neonatal care, simply did not survive long enough after birth to develop NEC. The same can be said about the second biggest group affected, namely babies with congenital heart disease, without modern medical and surgical care these babies died before they could contract NEC. Less than a century ago, these conditions were uniformly fatal and hence NEC did not exist as an identifiable disease prior to the twentieth century.

Since the late 1960s there has been a growing body of literature on this disease. We know a lot about NEC. There is still a lot that we do not know. The pathogenesis is complicated and multifactorial. We have made some strides in prevention but it remains a common disease in neonatal units. At the time of writing, treatment options are still very limited: NEC treatment remains supportive only with no specific therapeutic interventions. Outcomes remain essentially the same as they did

I. Jones, *Necrotising Enterocolitis in Clinical Practice*, In Clinical Practice, https://doi.org/10.1007/978-3-031-64148-0_1

three decades ago. This is in stark contrast to neonatology as a whole, where the progress that has been made it truly remarkable. Since the routine use of surfactant, the majority of pre-term infants survive and most do so without major disability. Mortality in preterm babies from respiratory disease continues to fall. As it does so, the proportion of neonatal death due to NEC grows.

Whilst this book is not intended to be an all-encompassing, comprehensive text it does cover all aspects of NEC: from definition of the disease, to the current understanding of the pathophysiology, to diagnosis, management, outcomes and potential future treatment options that offer some hope of better outcomes. In the third decade of the twentieth century, still a quarter of babies with NEC die and many of the survivors have life-long morbidity. This text is aimed at doctors, nurses and allied healthcare professionals with an interest in neonatal care. This will include neonatology specialists and paediatric surgeons. The purpose here is to bring together what is a large body of literature in a way that is accessible and concise. Readers should gain a good understanding of NEC and how to manage it and be much better placed to read new evidence and assimilate future therapeutic innovations in NEC management.

Chapter 2
History of Necrotising Enterocolitis

Contents

Abstract Necrotising enterocolitis emerged as a disease entity as neonatal care became established as a sub-specialty of paediatrics. By the mid-1980s, the key features of this disease were identified and broadly accepted. Management with antibiotics and surgery for the most severe cases became routine.

The introduction of routine surfactant use revolutionised neonatal care in the 1990s and many smaller, more premature babies survived than had done previously. In this context, NEC became both more common and more significant; fewer babies dying from respiratory problems has meant that NEC is now responsible for a higher proportion of deaths.

In the early part of the twentieth century, outcomes for neonates across the board have continued to improve but NEC treatment and prognosis has hardly changed at all.

Keywords Early descriptions of NEC · Historical cases of NEC · Development of NEC diagnosis · Evolution of NEC treatment · Milestones in NEC research Historical perspectives on NEC etiology · NEC epidemiology over time · Changes in NEC incidence · NEC in neonatal medicine history · Historical controversies in NEC management · NEC awareness and recognition through history · Historical advancements in NEC prevention strategies · NEC outbreaks or clusters in history NEC-related historical medical discoveries or breakthroughs · NEC-related historical medical literature or documents

I. Jones, *Necrotising Enterocolitis in Clinical Practice*, In Clinical Practice, https://doi.org/10.1007/978-3-031-64148-0_2

2.1   Introduction

Most human diseases known today were known in antiquity. There is ample documentation of cancer and infectious disease across civilisations. Medical advancement over the last few hundred years was for the most part an accelerating understanding of the pathophysiology of diseases. New diseases were identified but most of them already existed. Conversely NEC is a genuinely modern disease, it emerged in the middle of the twentieth century as neonatal care developed and mortality for the most vulnerable infants fell dramatically. Effectively there was a new population of human infants at risk of this new disease that had not existed before and hence NEC emerged as a phenomenon of neonatal units.

A PubMed search in 2024 on the term "necrotising enterocolitis" will return nearly 11,000 articles. Many of these are not focused on the neonatal disease and reflect the term being used descriptively rather than referring to the specific disease entity known as NEC. More striking though, is the pattern over time of publication on NEC. Throughout the 1960s, only 1–2 articles per year were published on NEC. For context, several hundred articles per year were published on "urinary tract infection" in the same decade and over 20,000 per year on "cancer." More specifically, looking at neonatal surgery, there were an average of 14 articles per year on "oesophageal atresia," 12 per year on "imperforate anus" and over 30 per year on "pyloric stenosis." Publication on NEC has grown exponentially since then but still there are fewer than 1000 articles per year being published.

The overall purpose of this text is to pull-together this literature into a coherent story of what is known and the key uncertainties and possible future directions for managing this devastating disease. Understanding the history of NEC is to some-extent a matter of interest rather than being directly relevant to clinical practice. However, understanding NEC in the context of its history aids understanding of this disease and why, despite impressive progress in our understanding of the pathophysiology of NEC, there remain so many gaps in our understanding. It also helps to understand how we arrived at various theories and approaches to NEC as well. In this chapter we will examine the earliest documented cases, the emergence of NEC as a recognised phenomenon in neonatal units and how the lack of progress made in NEC stands in stark contrast to the immense progress in neonatal outcomes overall.

2.2   First Documented Description

Charles-Michel Billard was born in 1800 in the Loire region of France. In the 1820s he worked in Paris, then the world centre of academic medicine [1]. In January 1826, he became *élève intern* at the Hôpital des Enfants-Trouvés [Hospital for Foundling Children]. There Billard worked under Dr. J.F Baron (1782–1849), who emphasised the importance of autopsy examination in the study of pathophysiology. In 1828 he published *A Treatise on the Diseases of Newborn and Suckling Infants*, based on his clinical experience [2]. This is a remarkable work of detailed clinical and pathological observations. It includes descriptions of neonatal conditions such as duodenal atresia, small bowel atresia and neonatal jaundice. Anyone with an interest in neonatal medicine would recognise so much of what Billard describes.

Given his brilliance for observation and detailed description it is not surprising that he can also be credited with the first known description of NEC. In 1823, he described 'gangrenous enterocolitis' in a 'weak infant with infection, inflammation and necrosis of the gastrointestinal tract.' [3].

The term 'Necrotising Enterocolitis'—as a specific disease entity—is generally credited to Mizrahi et al. over a hundred and forty years after Billard's first description, when they used the term to describe a clinical syndrome consisting of 'vomiting, abdominal distention, gastrointestinal bleeding, and shock in premature infants' in 1965 [4]. The previous year, the same group (as Berdon et al.) had published a report of 21 infants (out of over 2000 over 10 years) who were initially well at birth before developing enterocolitis. They also used the term 'necrotising enterocolitis' and asserted that multiple case reports of 'neonatal appendicitis,' 'colitis,' 'ileitis,' 'peritonitis,' or 'pneumotosis intestinalis' were most likely the same disease: NEC [5].

2.3 Emergence of the Disease Entity

Billard's experience of medicine in the newborn was ground-breaking but a world away from modern neonatology. He was able to make key and insightful observations but only on the basis of post-mortem examination. In the latter half of the twentieth century, neonatology was born as a subspecialty of paediatrics and as a consequence babies whose prognosis would previously have been entirely hopeless began to survive. It is in this context that it began to become clear that there was an intestinal condition to which premature babies were especially vulnerable. In 1974, a paper with the title "Necrotizing enterocolitis. An emerging entity in the regional infant intensive care facility" was published, indicating that by that point, neonatal units were well aware of this disease [6].

2.3.1 Neonatology: The Birth of a New Subspecialty

The term 'neonatology' was first coined by Alexander Schaffer in 1960 and in the following decade and a half, the sub-specialism of paediatrics became recognised [7]. The first neonatal unit in the USA was opened in 1965. This was not the earliest such unit though, as Southmead Hospital in Bristol, in England opened its eight bed unit for premature babies in 1946 [8]. Throughout the 1960s and 1970s the speciality evolved rapidly, underpinned by excellent scientific work. The key to neonatal care was the use of incubators and meticulous aseptic nursing. Staphylococcal infection was a particular problem in the early days.

Incubators themselves have a very odd history. The concept that some sort of container to allow effective thermoregulation for a human neonate is a relatively obvious one in a world where such devices already exist for chicks. Staphane Tarnier, an obstetrician is credited with the first working device which he put in to clinical use in the Paris Maternity Hospital in 1880. Martin Couney took the latest version of this device to the World Exposition in Berlin in 1896. Couney decided that it would be best demonstrated by including six live human neonates. He named his exhibit *Kinderbrutanstalt*—"the child hatchery" [9]. This very rapidly became a massive tourist attraction and a phenomenon of the age. Reportly the Kinderbrutanstalt was celebrated in comic songs and music hall jokes. This display was subsequently replicated at the Victorian Era Exhibition in 1897 in London. A Lancet editorial described the set up in detail and noted the potential for reducing mortality in prematurely born or 'delicate' infants [10]. Despite this, there was no wide scale adoption of incubators in clinical practice. These exhibitions were a huge financial success and subsequently Couney set up an exhibition on Coney Island in New York and at fairs across the USA. The babies in question were mostly considered 'weaklings' who would not survive but Courney managed to return a remarkable 85% of these babies to their parents [11]. The New York show closed in 1943. Whilst the ethical route by which the role of incubators in the care of premature babies was proven is far from ideal, unquestionably Couney had proven their value and laid the ground work for modern neonatology.

In the 1960s the notion of a specialist nursery for premature babies became fully established, building on the work done throughout the late 1940s and 1950s. Whilst much of the care was rudimentary by modern standards, and the gestation limit of viability was very different, for the first time there was a population of premature infants being cared for and surviving. It is, of course, in this context that the new disease of NEC began to be seen.

2.4 From Mizrahi to Bell: How We Began to Define the Disease

As the care of premature neonates developed and neonatology became a recognised sub-speciality of paediatrics, NEC emerged. Mizrahi's description of NEC in the early 1960s coined the term [4] and in 1978, Bell et al. [12] published a seminal paper on NEC. These are the key points in the discovery of this disease. Bell et al. suggested a clinical staging system for NEC that came to be known as the Bell Classification. They noted that a decade of study had begun to identify various factors that were associated with NEC but a lack of agreement on definitions, made comparison between reports extremely challenging. It is somewhat disappointing that so much of the literature in the following decades decry the same issues hampering progress.

Bell's classification was not meant to be used as a way of defining the disease—it was aimed at rationalising clinical management—but perhaps inadvertently, it has come to define the disease. Although in terms of describing the disease, it actually changed very little from Berdon's and Mizrahi's description;

> Usually weighing under 1,500 grams at birth, the babies showed a similar clinical pattern. They seemed well during the first forty-eight to seventy-two hours of life with no signs of respiratory distress or fever, and feedings were well tolerated. Following this variable period of well-being, delayed gastric emptying, bile-tinged emesis and gastric residue, and mild to severe abdominal distention developed; blood-streaked stools were then passed, though actual diarrhea was uncommon. Despite vigorous supportive and antibiotic therapy, the usual picture was one of deterioration with apneic spells, jaundice, shock, and death. [5]

Throughout that period, several case reports, case series and basic science studies were published as the disease entity that is NEC came to be recognised as an inevitable feature of neonatal practice.

In 1986, Walsh and Kleigman [13] published a broad review of NEC. Included in this paper was a stratification of NEC which built on the Bell Classification. This *modified*-Bell classification is still the most-widely used system in NEC [14].

Walsh and Kleigman's paper shows where the understanding of NEC had got to by that point. The introduction begins like this:

> Necrotizing enterocolitis (NEC) continues to be the most serious and most frequent gastro-intestinal disorder seen in neonatal intensive care units (NICU). The disease is characterized by signs of sepsis in addition to multiple gastrointestinal disturbances ranging from abdominal distention, bilious emesis, and hematochezia to intestinal perforation, peritonitis, and shock

They also report that the highest incidence of NEC is in babies weighing less than 1500 g, where it approaches 12% and that the US Centre for Disease Control and Prevention (CDC) data had suggested a mortality of 40% at the time.

They list 21 known risk factors for NEC:

 1. *Prematurity*
 2. *Perinatal asphyxia*
 3. *Respiratory distress syndrome (RDS)*
 4. *Umbilical catheterization*
 5. *Hypothermia*
 6. *Shock*
 7. *Hypoxia*
 8. *Patent ductus arteriosus (PDA)*
 9. *Cyanotic heart disease*
10. *Polycythemia*
11. *Thrombocytosis*
12. *Anemia*
13. *Exchange transfusion*
14. *Congenital gastrointestinal anomalies*

15. *Chronic diarrhea*
16. *Non-breast milk formula*
17. *Nasojejunal feedings*
18. *Hypertonic formula*
19. *Too much formula-too fast*
20. *Hospitalization during epidemic*
21. *Colonization with "necrogenic" bacteria*

They noted that 90% of the cases are in premature babies and the vast majority (at least 95%) had been enterally fed.

They also summarised very nicely the literature in terms of the understanding of NEC pathophysiology at that point:

> It is hypothesized that NEC is the final common response of the immature gastrointestinal system to potentially multiple injurious factors. In addition, the final mucosal pathology may be the result of simultaneous events that produce synergistic damage. Mechanisms of mucosal injury that have been implicated to be important in the pathogenesis of NEC, include gastrointestinal and immunologic immaturity, ischemia, colonization by and subsequent invasiveness of pathogenic enteric bacteria, isolated intestinal bacterial overgrowth, excess bacterial substrate, and immunologic injury from milk protein allergy.

Those words seem very prescient as the data accumulated in the decades since further support the hypotheses put forward here. Most of those risk factors listed are still undoubtedly relevant to the development of NEC. Very recent data suggests that the rate of feed advancement and the osmolality of feeding is not a risk for NEC but otherwise the list is comprehensive and supported by up-to-date data. The pathophysiology of NEC, or more specifically, the *pathogenesis* is described in detail in Chap. 5. It begins with looking at each of these risk factors and how they interact to cause the disease. Our understanding of NEC is built on this work.

It is fair to say that by the mid-1980s, the disease entity of NEC, as we understand it today, was established and acknowledged by neonatologists and surgeons. The biggest change since then is with the neonatal population. At this point very few of the babies with a birthweight less than 1000 g survived (around 10–15%). Similarly, only a third of those born between 1000 and 1500 g survived, whether they got NEC or not [15].

2.5   The Post-surfactant Era

A key concept in understanding the pathophysiology of NEC is that the premature intestine is not well-suited to ex-utero life. Put simply, in the foetus, the intestine has no role in absorption of nutrients and has very limited function. This mismatch between the need for the intestine to provide function once the baby is born and it's unsuitability to the task is undoubtedly key to the development of NEC.

The same can also be said for other organ systems, especially the lungs. The lungs have no role in gas exchange in utero and the immaturity of the lungs is a major cause of morbidity and mortality in babies born prematurely. As neonatal care developed, respiratory failure was a leading cause of mortality and morbidity, along with sepsis. It remains true that these—along with NEC—are the main challenges in the care of premature babies today.

In 1959, at the Montreal Pediatric Conference, Respiratory distress syndrome (RDS) was defined [8] (although controversy persists about the precise definition). RDS is characterised by acute respiratory distress: dyspnoea; trachypnoea; apnoeas and cyanosis, in premature neonates.

In the 1950s, it was shown that surfactant deficiency was the cause of RDS [16]. Pulmonary surfactant is produced by Type II pneumocytes and is vital for reducing the surface tension and allowing the lungs to expand. Production begins at 24 weeks completed gestation, but continues to mature until term. Hence the risk of RDS is inversely proportional to gestation. In the 1980s, the first studies were published on effective use of surfactant in human patients and since the 1990s it has become routine practice. As a consequence, mortality for babies born before 29 weeks fell by 60–73% virtually overnight [17]. Figure 2.1 shows the overall survival for babies with birthweights less than 1500 g from 1960 to 2015. For the smallest babies survival increased more than tenfold from less than 7% to over 70%. This longitudinal dataset is from Korea. European and North American outcomes are probably slightly better overall. However, this graph beautifully demonstrates the improvement in outcomes for premature neonates overall.

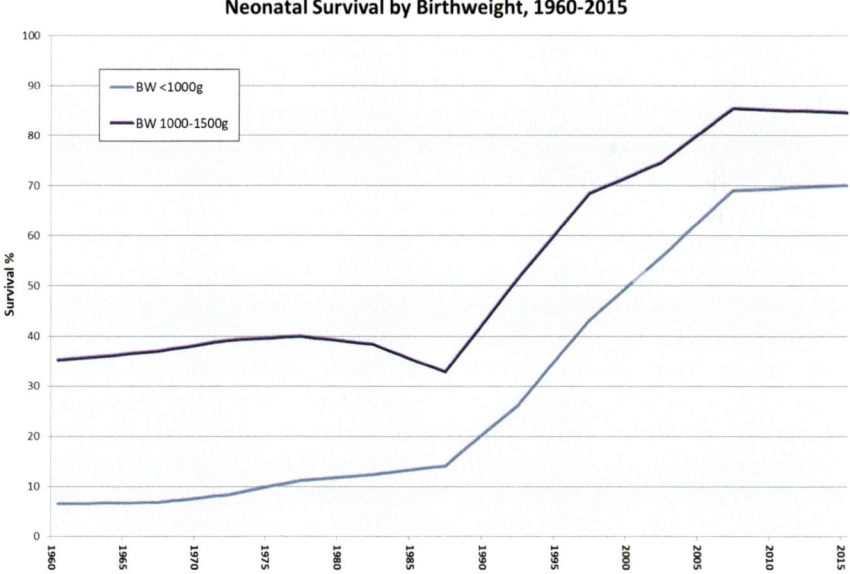

Fig. 2.1 Neonatal survival to discharge by birthweight 1960–2015. Based on Shim et al. [15]. The steep increase in survival corresponds with the introduction of tracheal-tube administered surfactant in the study population

This was a huge step-change in neonatal care, such that it is common in the literature to find the phrase 'post-surfactant era' indicating how big a step-forward this was. In the first decade of the twenty-first century, neonatal mortality continued to fall (with improved ventilatory strategies and the routine use of antenatal steroids and other step-wise improvement in neonatal care) [18].

This has important implications for NEC risk and management. The population of premature babies is increasing—as more survive the earliest weeks, meaning that the population at risk of NEC is increasing. At the same time, mortality from other causes is falling and therefore NEC is responsible for a rising proportion of neonatal deaths. One such study from the US shows that overall mortality for extremely premature infants (born at less than 29 weeks gestation) fell from 275 per 1000 live births in 2000–2003 to 258 per 1000 live births in 2008–2011. In the same time periods, death from respiratory causes fell from 83 per 1000 to 68 per 1000. Deaths attributed to NEC increased from 23 per 1000 to 30 per 1000. To put that another way, over the course of a decade, NEC went from being the primary cause of death in 8% of extremely premature neonates who died to being responsibly for 11% of deaths in this group. Moreover, there was an overall rise in mortality due to NEC as well as this rise in the proportion of deaths in neonates due to NEC [18].

2.6 Necrotising Enterocolitis: The State of the Art

It is tragically true to say that outcomes for NEC remain largely unchanged in the last three decades. There is still not a complete consensus on the definition of NEC. There has been a large amount of research on the pathophysiology of NEC but it would be a stretch to claim we have a complete picture of how the disease is caused. Certainly there is similarly no consensus on this point. There is a lot of research interest in the prevention of NEC as well as treatment. In essence, preventing NEC is very simple: simply prevent premature birth and that would take care of 90% of cases! Sadly that, for the moment at least, continues to be a forlorn hope. It is sobering to note that in a symposium for Child Health Day by the American National Institute of Child Health and Human Development in 1985, one speaker, reflecting on the remarkable progress made, stated *"Perhaps the next 30 years will bring about an equally miraculous decline in the incidence of low birth weight and its attendant problems."* [19] Those 30 years and more have passed and premature birth so far remains an unsolved problem and as such, it seems very unlikely that we will see a consequential reduction in NEC rates. It is also true that the treatment options described by Walsh and Kleigman in 1986 are mostly the same as how NEC is treated today [13].

The following chapters are dedicated to the current state of the art with NEC. Chapter 3 provides a definition of NEC, Chap. 4 examines the current epidemiology and Chap. 5 is a complete overview of what is known and what is unknown about the pathophysiology. Chapter 6 is dedicated to the prevention of NEC, whilst

Chap. 7 discusses the clinical management. Chapter 8 is dedicated specifically to surgical decision-making in NEC and Chap. 9 lays out the current data on short and long-term outcomes. Chapter 10 is dedicated to the future of NEC management: the potential new clinical interventions may become part of NEC prevention and treatment in the future.

References

1. Shulman S. Charles-Michel Billard, an overlooked pediatric pioneer. Hektoen Int; 2020.
2. Billard C. A treatise on the diseases of infants, founded on recent clinical observations and investigations in pathological anatomy made at the Hospice des Enfans-Trouvés. 1828. (English translation available in Welcome Collection: https://wellcomecollection.org/works/n7xdvhg8).
3. Sharma R, Hudak ML. A clinical perspective of necrotizing enterocolitis: past, present, and future. Clin Perinatol. 2013;40(1):27–51. https://doi.org/10.1016/j.clp.2012.12.012.
4. Mizrahi A, Barlow O, Berdon W, Blanc WA, Silverman WA. Necrotizing enterocolitis in premature infants. J Pediatr. 1965;66:697–705.
5. Berdon W, Grossman H, Baker D, Mizrahi A, Barlow O, Blanc W. Necrotizing enterocolitis in the premature infant. Radiology. 1964;83:190–4. https://doi.org/10.1148/83.5.879.
6. Roback SA, Foker J, Frantz IF, Hunt CE, Engel RR, Leonard AS. Necrotizing enterocolitis. An emerging entity in the regional infant intensive care facility. Arch Surg 1974;109(2):314–9.
7. Philip A. The evolution of neonatology. Pediatr Res. 2005;58(4):799–815. https://doi.org/10.1203/01.PDR.0000151693.46655.66.
8. Christie DA, Tansey EM. Origins of neonatal intensive care in the UK. London: The Wellcome Trust Centre for the History of Medicine; 1998.
9. National Institutes of Health. Neonatal intensive care—a history of excellence. A symposium commemorating child health day. 1985. https://neonatology.net/pdf/nic.nih1985.pdf.
10. The use of incubators for infants. Lancet. 1897:1490–1.
11. Barry RR. Coney Island's Incubator Babies. 2018. https://daily.jstor.org/coney-islands-incubator-babies/.
12. Bell MJ, Ternberg JL, Feigin RD, Keating JP, Marshall R, Barton L, Brotherton T. Neonatal necrotizing enterocolitis. Therapeutic decisions based upon clinical staging. Ann Surg. 1978;187(1):1–7.
13. Walsh MC, Kliegman RM. Necrotizing enterocolitis: treatment based on staging criteria. Pediatr Clin N Am. 1986;33(1):179–201.
14. Patel R, Ferguson J, McElroy S, Khashu M, Caplan M. Defining necrotizing enterocolitis: current difficulties and future opportunities. Pediatr Res. 2020;88(Suppl 1):10–5. https://doi.org/10.1038/s41390-020-1074-4.
15. Shim J, Jin H, Bae C. Changes in survival rate for very-low-birth-weight infants in Korea: comparison with other countries. J Korean Med Sci. 2015;30(Suppl 1):S25–34. https://doi.org/10.3346/jkms.2015.30.S1.S25.
16. Avery M, Mead J. Surface properties in relation to atelectasis and hyaline membrane disease. AMA J Dis Child. 1959;97(5, Part 1):517–23. https://doi.org/10.1001/archpedi.1959.02070010519001.
17. Dance A. Survival of the littlest: the long-term impacts of being born extremely early. Nature. 2020;582:7810. https://doi.org/10.1038/d41586-020-01517-z.
18. Patel RM, Kandefer S, Walsh MC, Bell EF, Carlo WA, Laptook AR, et al. Causes and timing of death in extremely premature infants from 2000 through 2011. N Engl J Med. 2015;372(4):331–40. https://doi.org/10.1056/NEJMoa1403489.
19. NIH. Neonatal intensive care a history of excellence a symposium commemorating child health day. 1985. https://neonatology.net/pdf/nic.nih1985.pdf.

Chapter 3
Definition of Necrotising Enterocolitis

Contents

Abstract Necrotising enterocolitis is an acquired condition seen primarily in premature infants that is characterised by intestinal wall inflammation leading to necrosis and potentially perforation. It most often presents with feed intolerance, systemic instability and abdominal distension. In the context of an unwell premature infant, pneumotosis intestalis on abdominal x-ray is pathopneumonic for NEC. The modified Bell staging system is the most widely used diagnostic criteria for NEC.

Clinically, a baby presenting with signs and symptoms, consistent with Bell Stage I should, initially, at least, be treated as NEC. From a research perspective, for most studies, it is more appropriate to only include babies meeting the criteria for Bell Stage IIa or higher.

© The Author(s), under exclusive license to Springer Nature
Switzerland AG 2024

I. Jones, *Necrotising Enterocolitis in Clinical Practice*, In Clinical Practice,
https://doi.org/10.1007/978-3-031-64148-0_3

Keywords Neonatal gastrointestinal disorder · Bowel necrosis · Intestinal inflammation · Acute necrotising enterocolitis · Premature infants and NEC Definition of NEC in newborns · NEC diagnosis criteria · Bell's staging criteria for NEC · Clinical signs of NEC · Radiological findings in NEC · Pathophysiology of NEC · Epidemiology of NEC · Risk factors for NEC · NEC in neonatal intensive care units · NEC in full-term infants · NEC in premature babies · NEC and gut microbiota · NEC and enteral feeding · NEC complications and outcomes

3.1 Introduction

Perhaps surprisingly, the exact definition of NEC remains controversial. There are several reasons for this, including the multifactorial nature of the pathophysiology (which is discussed in detail in Chap. 5) The fact is, that premature babies can become unwell for several reasons and the presenting features of NEC are often the same as (or very similar to) those seen in babies who have developed sepsis or some other diagnosis.

There are further debates about whether the 'NEC' that is seen in term babies with cardiac disease should be considered as the same entity as the disease we know as 'NEC' in premature babies.

This kind of uncertainty about the exact nature of a disease entity is actually not uncommon in medicine and deciding which patients fit with a particular diagnosis, or which criteria to use to define a particular diagnosis is seen in several other contexts, such as inflammatory bowel disease and chronic obstructive airways disease.

Therefore, for both clinical practice and research, we need a frame of reference to work with; some kind of diagnostic criteria that enables clinical decision-making and research on prevention, treatment and outcomes. It is important to note that the diagnostic criteria one uses clinically may not be the same as that which is used for research purposes. This is true in the case of NEC whereby the Bell Staging system (Sect. 3.3) provides an inclusive criteria for which babies to treat as NEC and a more exclusive criteria for research purposes. The Bell system is the best-known and most-widely used system but there are several others. This is discussed further in Sects. 3.3 and 3.4.

3.2 A Working Definition of NEC

Necrotising enterocolitis is an acquired condition seen in neonates that is characterised by bowel inflammation and necrosis and translocation of gas-forming bacteria into the bowel wall. The bowel injury can range from mucosal alone to full thickness necrosis and perforation. It can be present in an isolated area of both the small and large bowel or affect large segments of bowel or even the entire intestine (NEC Totalis). NEC can also result in damage to multiple other organ systems, as it can trigger a large systemic inflammatory response.

This definition describes and encompasses the disease entity that is NEC. There are several key points in here that are worth highlighting:

1. NEC is an *acquired* condition. It is not congenital. There is some debate about exact timings but in general, it is a disease of the second week of ex-utero life onwards.
2. The pathological features of NEC are intestinal inflammation and necrosis. This is nicely demonstrated by operative findings and pathological specimens. Whatever else is going on with NEC pathophysiology, there is a common end pathway of intestinal necrosis.
3. The role of bacterial infection in NEC in well-established and it is known that the cardinal feature of NEC of pneumotosis intestalis is due to gas-forming bacteria that have invaded the intestinal wall.
4. The injury of NEC is progressive. On the milder end of the scale, the injury is to the mucosa alone and at the other end of the scale, full thickness injury (involving every layer of the bowel wall) leading to perforation, is seen.
5. The disease can affect small areas of the intestine or can be very extensive. NEC is seen in both the small and large bowel. It is most common in the terminal ileum in premature neonates.
6. NEC is associated with systemic sepsis and multi-organ failure.

3.3 Modified Bell Staging

3.3.1 Bell Staging Criteria

In 1978, Bell et al. [1] proposed what came to be known as the Bell classification of NEC, later modified by Walsh and Kleigman [2]. The (modified) Bell classification remains the most widely-used diagnostic criteria for NEC [3]. The modified Bell classification is summarised in Table 3.1.

As described in Chap. 2, the clinical entity of NEC emerged as the advent of specialist neonatal care led to the survival of premature babies and by the late 1960s there was broad agreement that a new disease was clearly evident. Bell et al. [1] closely observed 48 patients diagnosed with NEC in two, related neonatal units, and identified three groups: Stage I—suspected NEC; Stage II—Definitive NEC; and Stage III—Advanced NEC.

The definition used for Stage I disease included systemic manifestations such as temperature instability, lethargy, apnoea, bradycardia and gastrointestinal manifestations of poor feeding, increasing gastric aspirates and vomiting which may or may not be bilious or contain blood and abdominal distention.

With Stage I disease, abdominal radiographs show distension with ileus (but no specific diagnostic features). A key concept that was noted, even in this original paper, is that many preterm infants will present with these features during their neonatal unit stay and yet not go on to develop further signs of NEC. In some cases

Table 3.1 Modified Bell Classification of NEC (Walsh and Kleigman [2])

Stage	Systemic signs	Abdominal signs	Radiographic signs	Treatment
(Ia) Suspected NEC	Temperature instability, apnoea, bradycardia, lethargy	Gastric retention, abdominal distention, emesis, haeme-positive stool	Normal or intestinal dilation, mild ileus	NPO, antibiotics × 3 days and review progress
(Ib) Suspected NEC	As Ia	Grossly bloody stool	As Ia	As Ia
(IIa) Definite NEC, mildly unwell	As above	Same as above, plus absent bowel sounds with or without abdominal tenderness	Intestinal dilation, ileus, pneumatosis intestinalis	NPO, antibiotics × 7 to 10 days
(IIb) Definite NEC, moderately unwell	Same as above, plus mild metabolic acidosis and thrombocytopenia	Same as above, plus absent bowel sounds, definite tenderness, with or without abdominal cellulitis or right lower quadrant mass	As IIa, plus portal venous gas +/− ascites	NPO, antibiotics × 14 days
(IIIa) Advanced NEC, severely ill, intact bowel	Same as IIa, plus hypotension, bradycardia, severe apnea, combined respiratory and metabolic acidosis, DIC, and neutropenia	Same as above, plus signs of peritonitis, marked tenderness, and abdominal distention	As IIa, plus ascites	NPO, antibiotics × 14 days, fluid resuscitation, inotropic support, ventilator therapy, paracentesis
(IIIb) Advanced NEC, severely ill, perforated bowel	As IIIa	As IIIa	Same as above, plus pneumoperitoneum	Same as IIIa, plus surgery

another diagnosis will become evident and it becomes clear over two days or so that something else is causing the symptoms. In others cases, the patient improves and no other diagnosis is apparent. In the absence of disease progression it is therefore impossible to determine how many of these really had NEC.

Bell defined Stage II disease as having the signs and symptoms of Stage I plus persistent occult or gross gastrointestinal bleeding and marked abdominal distension. Abdominal radiographs show significant intestinal distension with ileus and small bowel separation. Small bowel separation is the correct way to describe this radiological sign. It is seen with both bowel wall thickening and peritoneal fluid. Persistent bowel loops may be seen as well as pneumatosis intestinalis and portal venous gas. In the context of an unwell infant with abdominal signs, pneumatosis is pathopneumonic for NEC.

In this original classification, Stage III disease was defined as the features of Stage II disease with the addition of deterioration of vital signs, evidence of septic shock or marked gastrointestinal haemorrhage. Abdominal radiograph at this point, often shows a pneumoperitoneum in addition to the radiological features seen in Stage II.

3.3.2   Modified Bell Staging Criteria

In 1986, Walsh and Kleigman published a wide-ranging review on NEC and the state of the evidence at the time [2]. They proposed a modification to the Bell criteria adding an 'a' and 'b' to each Stage. This *modified* Bell criteria is the most common definition of NEC used in both clinical practice and research [3]. As Table 3.1 shows, Walsh and Kleigman recommended treatment based on the stage [2] It is perhaps most notable that literally decades later, the treatment is very similar.

3.4   Alternative Staging Systems and Definitions

Despite being the most-widely used criteria, the modified Bell staging system has important limitations. As discussed, the fact that many babies who meet the criteria for Stage I, often do not actually have NEC affects data analysis from a research perspective although usually it is appropriate to treat Bell Stage Ia/Ib babies as NEC. It is also the case that the various features including in the Bell staging are of varying sensitivity and specificity [3]. Accordingly, various other diagnostic criteria and staging systems have been proposed. These include the Vermont Oxford Network definition, the Centres for Disease Control and Prevention definition and the Gestational Age-specific Case definition for NEC developed by the UK Neonatal Collaborative Necrotising Enterocolitis Study Group.

3.4.1   Vermont Oxford Network (VON) Definition

The Vermont Oxford Network is an international collaboration of over 1200 centres that maintain large databases of neonates to support research and benchmark outcomes [4].

The VON criteria define NEC on post mortem, surgical findings or based on clinical and radiological features. The features used are all based on the Bell criteria but are more strictly applied. To make a diagnosis of NEC (in the absence of either surgery or post mortem), infants must have at least one of the defined clinical signs *and* one or more specific radiological finding. The clinical features used are: bilious gastric aspirate or emesis, abdominal distension or occult/gross blood in stool (no fissure). Pneumatosis intestinalis, portal venous gas and pneumoperitoneum are the specific radiological features used for the criteria.

3.4.2   Centre for Disease Control and Prevention (CDC) Definition

The Centre for Disease Control and Prevention is the United States' Government Health Agency with a particular focus on infectious diseases [5]. Their definition is very similar to the VON definition.

For the diagnosis of NEC by the CDC definition, infants must have at least one of the following clinical findings: bilious aspirates/vomiting/abdominal distention/blood in stools (with no anal fissure) *and* one or more relevant radiological feature: pneumatosis intestinalis/portal venous gas/pneumoperitoneum. The definition allows for equivocal radiological findings by including babies where the radiology is not clear cut but there is physician documentation of treatment of NEC with antimicrobials. In the same way as the VON criteria, these features are used to make a clinical diagnosis in babies who do not undergo surgery. In babies who have surgery the diagnosis of NEC is based on typical intra-operative findings such as pneumotosis and bowel necrosis.

3.4.3   United Kingdom Neonatal Collaborative Necrotising Enterocolitis Study Group (UKNC-NEC) Definition

The United Kingdom Neonatal Collaborative Necrotising Enterocolitis Study Group developed a points-based system with gestation-age specific cut-offs for diagnosis [6]. This system uses the same clinical features found in Bell's criteria or

Table 3.2   UKNC-NEC definition of NEC (Battersby et al. [6])

Clinical feature		Score
Pneumotosis intestalis		3
Blood in stool		2
Abdominal tenderness		1
Abdominal discolouration		1
One or more present:	Portal venous gas	
	Pneumoperitoneum	
	Fixed loop sign	1
Increased and/or bilious aspirates and abdominal distension		1
Total:		9
Diagnostic threshold by gestational age		
Gestation		
<26 weeks		2 or more
26–29 weeks, 6 days		2 or more
30–36 weeks, 6 days		3 or more
37 weeks or more		4 or more

the VON or CDC definitions. The distinctive difference being that it gives different weightings to each feature and the implications of each feature is different at different gestational ages. The scorings and diagnostic cut-off for each gestational group is summarised in Table 3.2. Intrinsically this system incorporates gestational age as a risk factor for NEC which is not the case with other systems. The authors reported a lower rate of classification error than other diagnostic systems, however it has not been more widely adopted.

3.4.4   2 of 3 Rule

The '2 of 3 Rule' is a system for the diagnosis of NEC that—as the name applies requires two of three specific features to be present, in the context of a classical clinical presentation. Thus the diagnosis is made in infants with abdominal distension and ileus or bloody stools with two of the following: pneumotosis and/or portal venous gas on radiograph or ultrasound at the time of diagnosis; persistent thrombocytopenia (<150,000 at 3 days) and infant age more consistent with NEC than SIP [3]. This is summarised in Table 3.3. This certainly has not had widespread acceptance but it is the only one of these systems that includes the platelet count in the diagnosis, which is perhaps surprising when thrombocytopenia is such a well-recognised feature of NEC

Table 3.3 '2 of 3 Rule' criteria for NEC diagnosis [3]

The 2 of 3 rule for diagnosing NEC		
Abdominal distension	Plus at 2 out of 3 of:	Pneumotosis and/or portal venous gas
AND		Persistent thrombocytopenia
Ileus or bloody stools		Infant age more consistent with NEC than SIP

3.5   'Cardiac NEC' Versus 'Neonatal NEC'

Babies born with congenital heart disease (CHD) are the second largest group to develop NEC after those born prematurely [7]. There is some debate in the literature as to whether 'cardiac NEC' is the same disease or should be considered as a separate entity. This is discussed further in Chap. 5 which examines the pathophysiology of NEC. The phenotype of NEC in cardiac babies is indeed slightly different to that which is seen in preterm babies with the colon being the most common site of disease (the terminal ileum is the most common site in premature neonates) [7]. However, babies with CHD and prematurity have the same common end-point of ischaemic necrosis of the intestine. Furthermore, babies born prematurely who also have CHD have a much higher risk of NEC than infants of the same gestation without CHD [8]. CHD confers a three to fourfold increase in the incidence of NEC in babies between 23 and 35 weeks gestation. The converse has also been demonstrated: one study (albeit with small numbers) showed a risk of NEC in term babies with CHD of 2% and 23% in babies with CHD who were also premature [9].

Therefore, whilst the pathogenesis differs, there are significant similarities in the presentation and management of these babies that supports considering it as part of the same disease process, whilst understanding the differences between the two sub-groups.

3.6   NEC and Spontaneous Intestinal Perforation

Spontaneous intestinal perforation (SIP), also known as focal intestinal perforation or isolated perforation is characterised by a single intestinal perforation in newborn infants. Most commonly it is seen in extremely low-birth weight infants and within the first week or two of life. Typically the perforation occurs in the terminal ileum.

Historically, SIP was considered as the same disease process as NEC but over time, evidence has shown it to be a clinical entity that is distinct from NEC [10]. Table 3.4 summarises the clinical differences between the two. Essentially SIP is a solitary perforation on the background of otherwise heathy intestine. Infants with SIP present earlier and do not have blood in their stools. There is also a clear histological difference between the two conditions. Chen et al. analysed the levels of the proteins HIF-1α and Glut-1 in surgical specimens from patients with both NEC and SIP. HIF-1α and Glut-1 are both markers of ischaemia. In patients with NEC both molecules were highly expressed whilst they were not seen in the SIP group [11].

Table 3.4 Differences between spontaneous intestinal perforation (SIP) and necrotising enterocolitis (NEC)

SIP	NEC
First week of life. Median age 7 days	After first week, median 15 days
No blood in stools	Bloody stools may be seen
Pneumoperitoneum	Pneumoperitoneum only in advanced disease
No Pneumotososis	Pneumatosis, portal venous gas
May or may not have systemic inflammatory response	Systemic inflammatory response
Normal intestine	Thickened bowel loops

3.7   Conclusion

The multifactorial nature of the pathogenesis of NEC, coupled with the variation in presenting features makes precise definitions difficult. However, from a clinical perspective, it is wise to treat babies who meet the criteria for Bell stage I or equivalent as having NEC (or suspected NEC) and therefore giving them a period of gut-rest and intravenous antibiotics before reviewing and deciding if an alternative diagnosis is appropriate. This is a safe practice but from a research perspective is problematic as it inevitably means that many infants who did not truly have NEC being included in the cohorts. As such, from a research perspective it is usually preferable to only include infants who meet the criteria for Bell stage IIa or above as definitively having NEC. Alternative diagnostic criteria may be more precise but are not widely used at present.

References

1. Bell MJ, Ternberg JL, Feigin RD, Keating JP, Marshall R, Barton L, Brotherton T. Neonatal necrotizing enterocolitis. Therapeutic decisions based upon clinical staging. Ann Surg. 1978;187(1):1–7.
2. Walsh MC, Kliegman RM. Necrotizing enterocolitis: treatment based on staging criteria. Pediatr Clin N Am. 1986;33(1):179–201.
3. Patel R, Ferguson J, McElroy S, Khashu M, Caplan M. Defining necrotizing enterocolitis: current difficulties and future opportunities. Pediatr Res. 2020;88(Suppl 1):10–5. https://doi.org/10.1038/s41390-020-1074-4.
4. Vermont Oxford Network. VON's public site. About us [Internet]. 2023. https://public.vtoxford.org/who-we-are-overview/. Accessed 26 Oct 2023.
5. CDC. About CDC. 2023. https://www.cdc.gov/about/. Accessed 28 Oct 2023.
6. Battersby C, Longford N, Costeloe K, Modi N. Development of a gestational age-specific case definition for neonatal necrotizing enterocolitis. JAMA Pediatr. 2017;171(3):256–63. https://doi.org/10.1001/jamapediatrics.2016.3633.
7. Maayan-Metzger A, Itzchak A, Mazkereth R, Kuint J. Necrotizing enterocolitis in full-term infants: case-control study and review of the literature. J Perinatol. 2004;24(8):494–9. https://doi.org/10.1038/sj.jp.7211135.

8. Kelleher S, McMahon C, James A. Necrotizing enterocolitis in children with congenital heart disease: a literature review. Pediatr Cardiol. 2021;42(8):1688–99. https://doi.org/10.1007/s00246-021-02691-1.
9. Natarajan G, Anne S, Aggarwal S. Outcomes of congenital heart disease in late preterm infants: double jeopardy? Acta Paediatr. 2011;100:1104–7. https://doi.org/10.1111/j.1651-2227.2011.02245.x.
10. Pumberger W, Mayr M, Kohlhauser C, Weninger M. Spontaneous localized intestinal perforation in very-low-birth-weight infants: a distinct clinical entity different from necrotizing enterocolitis. J Am Coll Surg. 2002;195(6):796–803.
11. Chen Y, Chang KT, Lian DW, Lu H, Roy S, Laksmi NK, et al. The role of ischemia in necrotizing enterocolitis. J Pediatr Surg. 2016;51(8):1255–61. https://doi.org/10.1016/j.jpedsurg.2015.12.015.

Chapter 4
Epidemiology of Necrotising Enterocolitis

Contents

Abstract Necrotising enterocolitis is a rare disease with an overall incidence reported in the range of 0.5–5.0 per 100,000 live births. This is a broad range and most likely the true incidence lies towards the lower end of this estimate when more precise definitions are used.

The incidence varies across the world with many countries and populations having a recognised higher incidence, whilst others have a lower incidence.

The vast majority of cases of NEC are found in babies born prematurely with an inverse relationship between gestational age and NEC risk: the most premature babies are at the highest risk. In term babies, NEC is almost always associated with specific risk factors, most commonly congenital cardiac disease.

In both premature babies and those born at term there are multiple risk factors that have been identified. The most important of these is enteral feeding and especially the type of feed. Cows' milk-based formula confers a much higher risk of NEC than human milk. Other factors include birth trauma, sepsis and anaemia.

© The Author(s), under exclusive license to Springer Nature
Switzerland AG 2024
I. Jones, *Necrotising Enterocolitis in Clinical Practice*, In Clinical Practice,
https://doi.org/10.1007/978-3-031-64148-0_4

Keywords NEC epidemiology · Incidence of NEC · Prevalence of NEC · NEC in premature infants · NEC in full-term infants · Risk factors for NEC · Gestational age and NEC · Birth weight and NEC · NEC in low birth weight infants · NEC in very low birth weight infants (VLBW) · NEC in extremely low birth weight infants (ELBW) · NEC by geographic region · NEC trends over time · NEC mortality rates · NEC morbidity rates · NEC and race/ethnicity · Gender differences in NEC incidence · Seasonal variation in NEC · Outcomes of NEC Long-term consequences of NEC

4.1   Introduction

NEC is a disease of prematurity. That is not to say that it is not seen in term infants. It is. However, it has long been recognised that over 90% of cases occur in infants born before 37 weeks completed gestation [1]. NEC in term infants is almost always associated with specific risk factors. Prematurity, as with all its biological phenomena and sequelae, is not a binary state. A baby born at 36 weeks and 3 days will have much more in common physiologically with a term baby than one born at 28 weeks for example. Moreover, gestational age is not entirely precise and hence much of the data we have in NEC is based on birth weight rather than gestational age. In simple terms though, the risk of NEC is inversely related to the number of weeks of completed gestation. The most premature babies have the highest risk of NEC and term babies have a much, much lower risk.

The incidence of NEC shows a big variation across the world, with some countries encountering NEC relatively frequently and others much less so. Implicitly, comparing developed countries to less developed ones means comparing across very different healthcare systems, but this variation is well-established in wealthier countries. The documented incidence of NEC lies within the range of 0.5–5 per 1000 live births [2].

4.2   Overall Incidence

As noted, estimates of the overall incidence of NEC vary widely. To some extent, this is a problem with the data. There remains insufficient consensus on the diagnostic criteria that should be used for NEC. The disease itself makes it challenging. What could be loosely termed 'early NEC' often has a very insidious onset. As Walsh and Kleigman [3] noted when they modified the Bell staging system, potentially a majority of babies who meet the criteria for Bell stage I (suspected NEC), do not in fact have NEC. In the original paper, Bell et al. [4] noted that most premature babies will have some of the features of NEC at some point. So, to some extent, it is inevitable that estimates of the incidence will vary. However, it is also true that the incidence of NEC varies between both countries and populations. A systematic review of NEC incidence in developed countries showed that among babies born before 32 weeks gestation there was a range of incidence between 2% and 7% and similarly a range of 5–22% in those born weighing less than 1000 g [5].

Based on data from a large cohort in neonatal units, Holman et al. 2006 [6] put the incidence of NEC in the USA at 1.1 per 1000 live births. Extrapolation from prospective UK data based on a survey of neonatal units would support an estimate of around 1000 UK cases each year [7] which corresponds to an incidence of around 1.4 per 1000 live births [8–10].

As noted, the true incidence of NEC varies. It occurs with higher frequency in North America, the UK and Ireland. It is much less common in Japan, Switzerland, and Austria [11]. This inevitably begs a question as to what is the cause of this variability? There are several plausible explanations. The populations are genetically diverse between these nations. Similarly environmental factors in the population, including socioeconomic factors differ between these countries. Undoubtedly there will be some variation in neonatal care practice. Added to which, whilst there is a big move to harmonise data collection methodology, differences still exist in the way NEC data is recorded. Which of these factors are responsible for the difference in incidence remains unclear.

There is some evidence from studies limited to the USA that a genetic predisposition is at least partly responsible for this difference. African American infants have a higher risk of NEC than Caucasians [12], even with correction for socioeconomic status. Similarly, twin studies support a genetic component of this risk [11]. In terms of which genes may be important for an increase risk of NEC, there is very limited data. The multifactorial nature of NEC pathophysiology means that there is a very large number of potential candidate genes [13], but at the time of writing, no specific genes have been identified.

4.3 Defining Prematurity: Gestational Age and Birth Weight

Normal human gestation is 38 weeks [14]. It takes an average of 268 days for a human to develop from a single cell to the point when ex-utero life begins. In general, the time of conception is difficult to be precise about for most people, whilst mothers do usually know—or have some idea—when their last menstrual period (LMP) occurred. For this reason, pregnancy has been traditionally counted from the first day of the mother's last period. Thus gestation is most commonly referred to as

Table 4.1 World Health Organisation definitions of prematurity [15] and low birth weight [16]

Neonatal definitions	
Prematurity	*Born before 37 completed weeks of gestation (defined from first day of last menstrual period)*
– Extremely premature	Less than 28 completed weeks of gestation
– Very premature	28 to 31 weeks, 6 days gestation
– Moderate to late premature	32 to 36 weeks, 6 days gestation
Birth weight	
Low birth weight (LBW)	<2500 g (1500–2499 g)
Very low birth weight (VLBW)	<1500 g (1000–1499 g)
Extremely low birth weight (ELBW)	<1000 g

a number of weeks out of a total of 40, adding on the average 14 days from the first day of menstruation to ovulation. In the 1970s it was demonstrated that dating based on ultrasonography during pregnancy was more reliable than the date of LMP and with the advent of routine scanning in developed countries, gestational dates are now primarily determined by measuring crown-rump length on ultrasound. The original terminology survived this technological revolution in obstetrics and continues to be used.

There is a (skewed) normal distribution around the 40 week mark and anything from 37 weeks, 0 days to 41 weeks, 6 days is considered term. The World Health Organisation defines prematurity therefore as any baby born before 37 weeks [15]. Premature babies are then further divided by their gestation into *moderate to late prematurity:* 32–37 weeks; *very premature*: 28–32 weeks and; *extremely premature*: less than 28 weeks (Table 4.1).

Even with the use of dating scans, gestational age can still be imprecisely measured. For this reason, much of the literature on neonates (including NEC) refers to birthweight rather than gestation. There is a large natural variation in birthweight but anything over 2.5 kg is considered normal. Low birthweight (LBW) refers to babies weighing between 1.5 and 2.5 kg; Very low birthweight (VLBW) describes babies weighing between 1 and 1.5 kg. Extremely low birth weight (ELBW) is defined as <1 kg.

Implicitly there is a strong correlation between gestational age and birth weight. With the exception of babies who are small for gestation age (SGA), the concept of LBW/VLBW/ELBW is analogous to the gestational age but birthweight's higher precision (and relative ease of collection of the data) means it is used more often in the NEC literature.

4.4 Prematurity and Necrotising Enterocolitis

Prematurity is the biggest risk factor for NEC, with an inverse relationship between risk and gestational age. In parallel with this there is an inverse relationship between the risk of NEC and birthweight. Fitzgibbons et al. (2009) provides excellent quantitative data on this relationship and is summarised in Table 4.2.

As Table 4.2 shows (in ELBW and VLBW infants) there is a clear inverse relationship between birth weight and the risk of developing NEC. However the effect of contracting NEC on overall mortality is greater in the larger infants. This is because the smallest of babies have the highest background mortality rate. Babies born weighing less than 750 g have around a one third mortality without contracting NEC and hence the additive effect of NEC is relatively small. Conversely, babies with a birth weight approaching 1500 g have a mortality rate of only 2.6% if they do not contract NEC and hence the effect on mortality of NEC is much greater.

These data are probably out of date in terms of the mortality as overall mortality for ELBW infants continues to fall. However, they demonstrate very nicely the inverse relationship between birthweight and NEC risk (and by implication the same inverse relationship between gestational age and NEC).

Birth weight and gestation are closely correlated, but at all gestations birthweight varies. As would be expected there is a normal distribution of weights for each completed week of gestation. A baby born above the 90th centile is considered large for gestational age and a baby born below the 10th centile, small for gestational age (SGA). The ranges vary between populations, but Table 4.3 shows some typical values based on the Fenton Pre-term Growth Charts [18].

The obvious correlation between birthweight and gestational age is evident in these data: A baby born prior to 28 weeks will tend to be under 1000 g and hence fit the category of ELBW. A baby who meets the criteria for SGA (small for their gestational age) is at higher risk of NEC than a baby with a normal birthweight for their gestation [19].

Table 4.2 NEC incidence and mortality by birth weight

NEC risk by birthweight					
				Mortality (%)	Adjusted mortality
Birth weight (g)	N	NEC	NEC risk (%)	NEC (non-NEC)	OR (95% CI)
501–750	13,050	1568	12.0	42.0 (34.0)	1.6 (1.4–1.8)
751–1000	16,993	1569	9.2	29.4 (10.7)	3.6 (3.1–4.2)
1001–1250	18,794	1063	5.7	21.3 (4.1)	7.5 (6.2–9.1)
1251–1500	22,970	758	3.3	15.9 (2.6)	9.9 (7.3–13.4)

Mortality for each birth weight is shown and in brackets, for babies born at the same weight who did not contract NEC (*based on* Fitzgibbons et al. [17])

Table 4.3 Updated Fenton Preterm Growth Chart for birthweight by gestation

Gestation (weeks)	Girls		Boys	
	Median	SGA	Median	SGA
22	509	427	533	447
23	580	473	615	509
24	656	515	693	547
25	742	564	790	602
26	842	614	901	660
27	946	671	1015	712
28	1072	738	1156	795
29	1222	842	1311	898
30	1391	974	1480	1035
31	1575	1120	1668	1221
32	1784	1337	1884	1416
33	2020	1527	2109	1633
34	2246	1752	2340	1839
35	2482	1991	2580	2079
36	2718	2197	2821	2297
37	2954	2416	3071	2529
38	3164	2639	3295	2755
39	3322	2807	3457	2925
40	3454	2938	3599	3059
41	3561	3026	3715	3153
42	3717	3159	3864	3249

Average indicated 50th centile and SGA (small for gestational age) is the limit of the 10th centile. A baby with a weight less than this figure would is SGA [18]
Further resources available from the website: https://live-ucalgary.ucalgary.ca/resource/preterm-growth-chart/preterm-growth-chart

4.5   Necrotising Enterocolitis in Term Infants

NEC is undoubtedly a disease of prematurity, that is sometimes seen in term babies. There is some controversy as to whether 'NEC' seen in term neonates should be considered as the same disease. This is discussed in detail in Chap. 5 but the risk factors that are associated with NEC in term babies are also associated with an increased risk of NEC in premature babies. Therefore even though it is arguably correct to think of NEC as a spectrum of diseases with multiple causes, there is at least significant overlap in the pathogenesis between term and pre-term NEC. It makes sense to consider it as a single disease with multiple, diverse causative factors.

There are several risk factors in term infants that have been implicated in the development of NEC, and it is vanishingly rare to see NEC in a term infant without such a risk factor. Identified risks include: low Apgar scores, birth asphyxia, sepsis, gastroschisis and congenital defects (such as cardiac or gastrointestinal anomalies) [20, 21].

Table 4.4 Risk factors for NEC in term infants

Feature	Developed NEC (n = 30)	Did not develop NEC (n = 5847)	NEC risk	p value
Congenital heart disease	27% (8)	5% (270)	2.9%	0.000
Polycythaemia	7% (2)	0.2% (13)	13.3%	0.003
Early-onset bacterial sepsis	13% (4)	2% (131)	3.0%	0.005
Birth weight (g)	2849 ± 581	3180 ± 594		0.010
Hypotension	27% (8)	13% (713)	1.1%	0.025
Endotracheal intubation	60% (18)	41% (2395)	0.7%	0.041

Based on Lambert et al. [20], the risk of NEC in a term neonate admitted to the neonatal unit was 30/5877 (0.51%). However, risk ratios (RR's) could not be calculated as the data did not report NEC risk in neonates without each specific feature. p-values (apart from birth weight) calculated using Fisher's Exact Test

Table 4.4 shows data from one study on NEC risk in term babies. These data would suggest a risk of NEC of approximately 0.5% for term babies that require admission to the neonatal unit. By definition therefore, this is within a sub-group with risk factors. The majority (60%) of the babies who developed NEC were already intubated and ventilated. Conversely only a minority of babies (0.7%) that were intubated for whatever reason developed NEC. Similarly, nearly a third of babies with congenital cardiac conditions developed NEC but the majority of the infants with heart conditions did not. The numbers are small in this series, but polycythaemia appears to be associated with a high NEC risk. A risk as high as 13% would mean these babies have an equivalent risk to the smallest preterm babies but polycythaemia itself is rare in term babies admitted to the neonatal unit.

4.5.1 Congenital Cardiac Disease and Necrotising Enterocolitis

In simple terms, NEC occurs in three groups of neonates: those born prematurely, those born with congenital heart disease (CHD) and others. Babies born with CHD are the second largest group and make up the majority of the 10% of cases that occur in term babies [22, 23].

CHD is an umbrella term and there is huge heterogeneity between difference congenital cardiac lesions. Within the whole spectrum of CHD, specific diagnoses and/or physiological states are associated with an increased risk of NEC. Hypoplastic left heart syndrome is associated with a nearly fourfold increase in NEC risk and Truncus or aortopulmonary window with a sixfold increase in NEC risk [24]. In the same data series, being born at a lower (but near-term) gestational age correlated with a fourfold increase in NEC risk. Episodes of low cardiac output or clinical shock also conferred a greater than sixfold increase in the risk of developing NEC.

4.5.2   Other Risk Factors in Term Infants

As noted above, the vast majority of babies who contract NEC are born prematurely and of the remaining 10%, most will have a congenital cardiac lesion. The small number of cases that occur in the remaining population are associated with a long list of potential risk factors. Because of the small numbers involved, there is limited data which makes quantifying these risk factors very difficult. Table 4.4 provides some quantitative data but only for a very limited number of factors because of the relatively small cohort used with only 30 cases of NEC among nearly 6000 term infants. The following is a list of risk factors that have been implicated in NEC in term infants (in addition to CHD) [25]:

- Maternal/antenatal factors:

  - Maternal hypertensive disease
  - HIV-positive mother
  - Placental insufficiency
  - Intrauterine growth restriction
  - Maternal illicit drug use

- Perinatal factors:

  - Perinatal asphyxia
  - Maternal infection
  - Umbilical catheters
  - Apgar score < 7 at 5 min

- Post Natal factors:

  - Polycythemia
  - Patent ductus arteriosus / Indomethacin use
  - Formula feeding
  - Exchange transfusion
  - Mechanical ventilation
  - Sepsis
  - Respiratory distress syndrome

- Other Factors:

  - Gastroschisis

4.6   Other Risk Factors for NEC in Premature Babies

There are a few additional risk factors that are applicable to premature babies which are not applicable to those born at term but the clear picture that emerges here is that when premature babies are exposed to the same risk factors that are associated with

NEC in term babies, they have an increased risk of NEC compared to babies of the same gestation who were not exposed to the same factors. This is the primary argument for not trying to separate out 'term-NEC' or 'cardiac-NEC.' The differences are important but ultimately the amount of overlap is very high and thus it is appropriate to consider all NEC as part of the same pathophysiology.

Below is a list of risk factors that have been implicated in NEC in premature babies. Note the similarity with the list for term babies [25] It should be noted that the strength of the evidence is far from uniform and it is debatable that all these factors are important and the relative importance of each of them is not entirely established.

- Antenatal factors

    - Intrauterine growth restriction (small for gestational age)
    - Chorioamnionitis
    - HIV-positive mother
    - Maternal cocaine use

- Perinatal factors

    - Perinatal asphyxia
    - Apgar score < 7 at 5 min

- Postnatal factors

    - Feeding

        - Formula feeding
        - Breast milk fortifier

    - H_2 blockers
    - Sepsis

        - Number of infections
        - Prolonged ($\geq$5 day) first course of antibiotics

    - Patent ductus arteriosus/Indomethacin treatment
    - Glucocorticoids and Indomethacin in first week of life
    - Mechanical ventilation
    - Morphine Infusion
    - Anaemia/blood transfusions

- Other factors

    - Black race

As noted, there are a lot of factors listed here. Some are almost certainly associations rather than having a causative relationship. A systematic review in 2022, included 52 different studies, totalling over 150,000 neonates provides some quantification of these risks [19]. Their meta-analyses concluded that antenatal factors such as premature rupture of membranes and gestational diabetes increased the risk

Table 4.5 Risk factors and odds ratios for developing NEC, *based on* Su et al. [19]

Risk factor	Odds ratio
Gestational diabetes	3.62
Premature rupture of membranes	3.81
Premature birth	5.63
Low birth weight	3.00
Small for gestational age	1.85
Congenital heart disease	2.73
Pneumonia	4.07
Septicaemia	4.34
Blood transfusion	3.08
Respiratory distress syndrome	2.12

of NEC. They showed that premature birth, low birth weight, being small for gestational age and congenital heart disease, were quantifiable risk factors for NEC as well as post-natal factors such as pneumonia, septicaemia, receiving a blood transfusion and respiratory distress syndrome (Table 4.5). This does not mean that the other suggested factors are not relevant but illustrates that the strength of evidence that exists for some factors is greater than others. Importantly, not every factor is considered in every study.

4.7   Location of NEC Within the Intestine

Necrotising enterocolitis is found throughout the intestine. The most common site of disease is within the terminal ileum [23]. Data from a large US database study shows that approximately 40% on infants who undergo surgery for NEC have disease limited to the small bowel whilst 18% will have only colonic disease [26]. There is also a difference between term babies with CHD disease and preterm babies with NEC. In babies with CHD, it is more common to find NEC in the colon only.

4.8   Conclusion

Incidence of NEC varies between populations and the reasons for this are multifactorial. Overall incidence is around 1–2 per 100,000 live births. The majority of cases of NEC occur in premature infants. NEC has an inverse correlation with gestational age and hence is most commonly seen in the smallest, most premature babies. In term babies, NEC is extremely rare in the absence of a clear risk factor. The most prominent of which is congenital cardiac disease. Enteral feeding, especially with cows' milk based formula feeds, sepsis, respiratory distress syndrome and the need for blood transfusion are also demonstrated risk factors for NEC.

References

1. Hall NJ, Eaton S, Pierro A. Royal Australasia of Surgeons Guest Lecture. Necrotizing enterocolitis: prevention, treatment, and outcome. J Pediatr Surg. 2013;48(12):2359–67. https://doi.org/10.1016/j.jpedsurg.2013.08.006.
2. Lin J, Nafday SM, Chauvin SN, Magid MS, Pabbatireddy S, Holzman IR, Babyatsky MW. Variable effects of short chain fatty acids and lactic acid in inducing intestinal mucosal injury in newborn rats. J Pediatr Gastroenterol Nutr. 2002;35(4):545–50.
3. Walsh MC, Kliegman RM. Necrotizing enterocolitis: treatment based on staging criteria. Pediatr Clin N Am. 1986;33(1):179–201.
4. Bell MJ, Ternberg JL, Feigin RD, Keating JP, Marshall R, Barton L, Brotherton T. Neonatal necrotizing enterocolitis. Therapeutic decisions based upon clinical staging. Ann Surg. 1978;187(1):1–7.
5. Battersby C, Santhalingam T, Costeloe K, Modi N. Incidence of neonatal necrotising enterocolitis in high-income countries: a systematic review. Arch Dis Child Fetal Neonatal Ed. 2018;103(2):F182–9. https://doi.org/10.1136/archdischild-2017-313880.
6. Holman RC, Stoll BJ, Curns AT, Yorita KL, Steiner CA, Schonberger LB. Necrotising enterocolitis hospitalisations among neonates in the United States. Paediatr Perinat Epidemiol. 2006;20(6):498–506. https://doi.org/10.1111/j.1365-3016.2006.00756.x.
7. Rees CM, Eaton S, Pierro A. National prospective surveillance study of necrotizing enterocolitis in neonatal intensive care units. J Pediatr Surg. 2010;45(7):1391–7. https://doi.org/10.1016/j.jpedsurg.2009.12.002.
8. Office for National Statistics: Births in England and Wales 2019 [Internet]. 2019. https://www.ons.gov.uk/peoplepopulationandcommunity/birthsdeathsandmarriages/livebirths/bulletins/birthsummarytablesenglandandwales/2019. Accessed 11 Dec 2020.
9. National Records of Scotland: Births 2019 [Internet]. 2019. https://www.nrscotland.gov.uk/statistics-and-data/statistics/scotlands-facts/births-in-scotland. Accessed 11 Dec 2020.
10. Northern Ireland Statistics and Research Agency: Births 2019 [Internet]. 2019. https://www.nisra.gov.uk/statistics/births-deaths-and-marriages/births. Accessed 11 Dec 2020.
11. Zani A, Pierro A. Necrotizing enterocolitis: controversies and challenges. F1000Res. 2015;4:F1000. https://doi.org/10.12688/f1000research.6888.1.
12. Llanos A, Moss M, Pinzòn M, Dye T, Sinkin R, Kendig J. Epidemiology of neonatal necrotising enterocolitis: a population-based study. Paediatr Perinat Epidemiol. 2002;16(4):342–9. https://doi.org/10.1046/j.1365-3016.2002.00445.x.
13. Cuna A, George L, Sampath V. Genetic predisposition to necrotizing enterocolitis in premature infants: current knowledge, challenges, and future directions. Semin Fetal Neonat Med. 2018;23(6):387–93. https://doi.org/10.1016/j.siny.2018.08.006.
14. Jukic A, Baird D, Weinberg C, McConnaughey D, Wilcox A. Length of human pregnancy and contributors to its natural variation. Hum Reprod. 2013;28(10):2848–55. https://doi.org/10.1093/humrep/det297.
15. Blencowe H, Cousens S, Oestergaard M, Chou D, Moller A, Narwal R, et al. National, regional, and worldwide estimates of preterm birth rates in the year 2010 with time trends since 1990 for selected countries: a systematic analysis and implications. Lancet. 2012;379(9832):2162–72. https://doi.org/10.1016/S0140-6736(12)60820-4.
16. Department of Nutrition for Health and Development WHO. Global nutrition targets 2025: low birth weight policy brief. Geneva: World Health Organization; 2018.
17. Fitzgibbons SC, Ching Y, Yu D, Carpenter J, Kenny M, Weldon C, et al. Mortality of necrotizing enterocolitis expressed by birth weight categories. J Pediatr Surg. 2009;44(6):1072–5.; ; discussion 5–6. https://doi.org/10.1016/j.jpedsurg.2009.02.013.
18. Fenton T, Kim J. A systematic review and meta-analysis to revise the Fenton growth chart for preterm infants. BMC Pediatr. 2013;13:59. https://doi.org/10.1186/1471-2431-13-59.
19. Su Y, Xu R, Guo L, Chen X, Han W, Ma J, et al. Risk factors for necrotizing enterocolitis in neonates: a meta-analysis. Front Pediatr. 2023;10:666507. https://doi.org/10.3389/fped.2022.1079894.

20. Lambert DK, Christensen RD, Henry E, Besner GE, Baer VL, Wiedmeier SE, et al. Necrotizing enterocolitis in term neonates: data from a multihospital health-care system. J Perinatol. 2007;27(7):437–43. https://doi.org/10.1038/sj.jp.7211738.
21. Oldham K, Coran A, Drongowski R, Baker P, Wesley J, Polley T. The development of necrotizing enterocolitis following repair of gastroschisis: a surprisingly high incidence. J Pediatr Surg. 1988;23(10):945–9. https://doi.org/10.1016/s0022-3468(88)80392-0.
22. Mukherjee D, Zhang Y, Chang DC, Vricella LA, Brenner JI, Abdullah F. Outcomes analysis of necrotizing enterocolitis within 11 958 neonates undergoing cardiac surgical procedures. Arch Surg. 2010;145(4):389–92. https://doi.org/10.1001/archsurg.2010.39.
23. Maayan-Metzger A, Itzchak A, Mazkereth R, Kuint J. Necrotizing enterocolitis in full-term infants: case-control study and review of the literature. J Perinatol. 2004;24(8):494–9. https://doi.org/10.1038/sj.jp.7211135.
24. McElhinney DB, Hedrick HL, Bush DM, Pereira GR, Stafford PW, Gaynor JW, et al. Necrotizing enterocolitis in neonates with congenital heart disease: risk factors and outcomes. Pediatrics. 2000;106(5):1080–7.
25. Gephart SM, McGrath JM, Effken JA, Halpern MD. Necrotizing enterocolitis risk: state of the science. Adv Neonatal Care. 2012;12(2):77–87.; ; quiz 8–9. https://doi.org/10.1097/ANC.0b013e31824cee94.
26. Zhang Y, Ortega G, Camp M, Osen H, Chang DC, Abdullah F. Necrotizing enterocolitis requiring surgery: outcomes by intestinal location of disease in 4371 infants. J Pediatr Surg. 2011;46(8):1475–81. https://doi.org/10.1016/j.jpedsurg.2011.03.005.

Chapter 5
Pathophysiology of Necrotising Enterocolitis

Contents

© The Author(s), under exclusive license to Springer Nature
Switzerland AG 2024
I. Jones, *Necrotising Enterocolitis in Clinical Practice*, In Clinical Practice,
https://doi.org/10.1007/978-3-031-64148-0_5

Abstract Necrotising enterocolitis is a multifactorial disease. We know that prematurity, enteral feeding (especially with cows' milk-derived formula), colonisation of the intestine with pathogenic bacteria and congenital cardiac disease are all risk factors for NEC.

Detailed studies have also shown that immunological dysfunction leads to intestinal inflammation and that ischaemia-reperfusion injury plays a part as well, resulting in ischaemic necrosis of the bowel.

NEC pathophysiology is best understood by the interaction of all these factors. Bacterial colonisation occurs prior to the onset of NEC but many babies will be colonised without going on to develop the disease. Formula feeds promote bacterial overgrowth. Bacterial invasion of the intestinal wall occurs and causes inflammation. The premature intestine does not regulate its blood flow properly, meaning that it is not always able to increase intestinal perfusion in response to feeding. The premature intestine is also more prone to inflammation than the term infant's. Inflammation increases the metabolic demand and can lead to relative ischaemia.

Once injury occurs, there is a vicious cycle as inflammation causes ischaemia which damages the intestinal wall and causes more inflammation. Breakdown in the intestinal barrier increases the risk of bacterial invasion. Bacterial invasion causes inflammation, ultimately resulting in ischaemic necrosis of the bowel. In severe cases, the infants become unwell with a systemic inflammatory response due to the severe inflammation and bowel perforation occurs leading to contamination of the peritoneum with intestinal contents.

Keywords NEC pathophysiology · Intestinal ischemia · Mucosal injury · Impaired gut barrier function · Inflammation in NEC · Intestinal microbiota dysbiosis Immature immune system in NEC · Hypoxia-reperfusion injury · Enterocyte apoptosis · Toll-like receptors in NEC · Cytokine cascade in NEC · Role of platelet-activating factor in NEC · Intestinal perfusion abnormalities · Role of enteral feeding in NEC pathogenesis · Role of formula feeding in NEC · Gut microbial colonization in NEC · Role of bacterial translocation in NEC · Genetic predisposition to NEC · Role of inflammation in NEC progression · Intestinal barrier dysfunction in NEC

5.1 Introduction

Since the disease entity of NEC emerged, there has been extensive research aimed at trying to understand the pathophysiology of NEC. This research comprises a broad sweep of clinical studies, epidemiological evidence and basic science research. All of which have built up the picture of the disease and added to our understanding. The purpose of this chapter is twofold. Firstly, to describe and assimilate the evidence that exists on NEC risk factors and pathogenesis. Secondly, to try to pull this evidence together into a coherent story of the disease that is Necrotising enterocolitis.

Any examination of the literature on NEC will show that there is not a consensus on the pathological processes involved. Inevitably, therefore, some of this will be speculative. However, for the most part, the differences seen in the literature are differences in emphasis only. Multiple factors are important in the development of NEC, and the evidence is clear on many of these factors. The controversy remains in how these factors interact to cause the disease and which are most important.

Chapter 3 explains the difficulties and challenges in defining NEC precisely. For the purposes of this text, the following definition is used:

> Necrotising enterocolitis is an acquired condition seen in neonates that is characterised by bowel inflammation and necrosis and translocation of gas-forming bacteria into the bowel wall. The bowel injury can range from mucosal alone to full thickness necrosis and perforation. It can be present in an isolated area of both the small and large bowel or affect large segments of bowel or even the entire intestine (NEC Totalis). NEC can also result in damage to multiple other organ systems as it can trigger a large systemic inflammatory response.

Whilst there remains some controversy around the exact definition of NEC and particularly around case-definition (i.e. which patients to include and which to exclude), that will inevitably make it more difficult to make progress in understanding the pathophysiology of the disease. Conversely, better understanding of the pathogenesis may lead to a clearer understanding of our definition of NEC.

This chapter will examine the evidence that has identified several different risk-factors for NEC. It will also look at multiple studies—both human and animal studies—that have investigated the pathogenesis of the disease and how these risk factors lead to intestinal injury.

Ultimately, a complete understanding of NEC must incorporate the multiple known risk-factors: it must incorporate how prematurity, enteral feeding, bacterial colonisation, immunological factors and localised hypoperfusion interact to result in intestinal inflammation and ultimately ischaemic necrosis of the bowel.

Sections 5.2, 5.3, 5.4, 5.5, and 5.6 discuss known risk factors for NEC in turn. However it is not correct to think of them separately as undoubtedly there is significant interaction between these factors. Indeed the pathogenesis is often due to a synergy between one or more of these factors that then results in NEC. This complex interaction has been, and remains, a challenge for the NEC research community. Conversely, each of the risk factors is an important starting point for investigating the causes of NEC and each tells us something important about the disease and is a way to begin to understand how the disease occurs and develops.

The focus of this chapter is the pathogenesis of NEC—how the disease occurs in the intestine. Severe NEC results in a systemic inflammatory response which leads to multi-organ failure and has an effect on the developing brain. The mechanisms by which systemic upset causes an injury to the developing brain is discussed in Sect. 9.4.

5.2   Prematurity

As already noted (Chap. 4), around 90% of cases of NEC occur in premature neonates [1]. Therefore, it is clear that prematurity is a key factor in the pathogenesis of NEC. Implicitly, there is something (or rather several 'things') about being born 'too-early' that makes babies vulnerable to this disease.

5.2.1   The Immature Intestine and NEC

Conceptually, it is not surprisingly that the premature gut is not well-adapted to ex-utero life. Post birth, the intestine is a vital organ; absorbing nutrients, maintaining a barrier against infection and maintaining electrolyte haemostasis. Increasingly there is evidence to show it has broader functions as well. The importance of the intestinal biome for overall health, including mental health is emerging with increasing evidence. Conversely, it has no known specific function prior to birth. The placenta provides the foetus with their nutrient requirements for metabolism and growth and provides the equivalent role of electrolyte haemostasis. There is no barrier function for the intestine in-utero as the whole foetus is within a sterile environment.

When babies are born prematurely, several of the organ systems are suddenly tasked with functions for which they are not yet fully developed. The lungs are probably the most critical of these organ systems. The cardiovascular system goes through major and very rapid changes at birth which include the closure of the ductus-arteriosus. It therefore is not surprising that the presence of a PDA (patent ductus arteriosus) is more common in premature babies compared to term infants. The kidneys' function prior to birth is significantly different to post birth and glomerular function is impaired at birth compared to an older infant, especially in the first 48 h of life. In each case, the function of these organs has in part or whole been carried out by the placenta up until birth. The intestine is no exception.

By 20 weeks gestation, the anatomical arrangement of the intestine is essentially complete and it is very similar to the term infant. However, the functional capability of the intestine remains underdeveloped [2]. There are multiple factors that make the intestine vulnerable to NEC which are discussed in the following sections but each of these is either, caused or exacerbated, by prematurity.

There is an inverse relationship between gestational age and the risk of developing NEC. In parallel there is an inverse relationship between birthweight and NEC risk. Whether gestational age or birth weight is the better measure of the maturity of an infant is debateable. This is partly due to the variation in estimates of gestational age and presumably due to natural variation in infants as well. The majority of the literature uses birthweight rather than gestational age, as it is easier to collect precise data but for our purposes here, the two are mostly analogous. Smaller, more premature babies are at a higher risk of NEC.

One UK study showed an NEC risk of 11% in babies born at 24 weeks, falling to 0.5% in infants born at 31 weeks. Table 4.2 shows the risk of NEC by birthweight up to 1500 g: 12% in babies between 500 and 750 g, falling to 3.3% in babies between 1250 and 1500 g [3]. The key concept here is that with each week of completed gestation, the intestine changes and the risk of NEC reduces. Over time the premature gut becomes more like the term infant's intestine and less prone to developing NEC.

As stated above, it is implicitly difficult to separate birth weight from gestational age but sub-group analysis in at-least two studies has shown that being small for gestational age (SGA) (i.e. a lower birth weight than would be expected for a specific gestational age) is an independent risk factor for NEC [4, 5]. Again, this probably indicates intestinal immaturity. It is well understood that under stress a developing foetus will often have asymmetric growth with the head (and therefore brain) preserved at the expense of other systems.

So, what is different about the premature gut that makes it vulnerable to this disease? The premature intestine has reduced motility. It only achieves the mature pattern of peristalsis from 35 weeks onwards [6]. This epitomises how the intestine is anatomically mature whilst not yet fully developed functionally. Reduced motility itself is likely to be a contributory factor, as it increases the risk of bacterial overgrowth and may well have other effects also.

Traditionally, the immune system has been divided into innate and acquired systems. The innate immune system includes many of the complex processes seen in the acquired immune system as well. It also encompasses physical barriers to infection such as the skin. The stomach and the pancreas contribute to this physical barrier and reduce the bacterial load on the small intestine. Gastric hydrochloric acid is bactericidal, as are pancreatic exocrine secretions [7]. Studies have shown that in premature infants, both gastric acid [8] and pancreaticobiliary secretions [9] have impaired production compared to what would be expected in a term neonate. In simple terms the oral route for bacteria to colonise the intestine is protected by these factors. In a premature baby this protection is not as effective as in a term neonate. Once beyond the stomach, colonisation of the intestine is impaired by other innate factors, Normal gut mucus is part of this process as it prevents adherence of bacteria to the intestinal wall. Mucus contains multiple factors that are important for preventing bacterial invasion. It has been shown experimentally that many of these factors are under-produced in the premature intestine. The intestinal mucus is made up of highly glycosylated protein referred to collectively as mucin. Mucin does not reach full production levels until 27 weeks of gestation [10], implying that any baby born before this point will have a reduced physical barrier throughout the bowel.

Within intestinal crypts are Paneth cells that produce multiple peptides including α-defensin and lysozyme-C [11], which have antimicrobial properties. Both the number of Paneth cells, and the production of α-defensin are reduced in human premature infants [12, 13]. The whole range of peptides produced by Paneth cells limit pathogen colonisation and invasion in the gut [13].

These differences go a long way to explaining why NEC is prevalent in preterm infants and not in term babies. They also show a kind of 'dose-effect' of prematurity: The more premature the baby—the fewer weeks of gestation completed, the less suited to ex-utero life is the intestine and therefore the higher the risk of NEC. However, notwithstanding these factors, the majority of premature infants do not get NEC. Several other factors are also important.

5.2.2   The Pathologenesis of Necrotising Enterocolitis in Term Infants: Is It the Same Disease?

If 90% of cases of NEC occur in premature babies then inescapably prematurity is very important in the pathogenesis of the disease but it does beg the question: what about the other 10%? Or to put it another way, if prematurity is necessary for the development of NEC, then one in ten of the cases we see would not happen. Prematurity alone cannot explain the onset of disease in this (not insignificant) minority of cases. Within the literature there has been significant debate about 'term-NEC.' Some argue that NEC should not be considered a single disease entity because of the multifactorial pathogenic pathways involved [14]. Following the logic of this argument, one could argue that term-NEC is in fact a different disease entity.

The risk factors for NEC in term infants are explored in Sect. 4.3 (Table 4.1). The most prominent of which is congenital cardiac disease but several others are also well documented.

An important counter argument to the complete separation of 'term NEC' is that when the same risk factors are seen in preterm infants, they have an increased risk of developing NEC compared to equivalent premature infants without those risk factors [15]. This suggests that whilst it is not a simple, single pathway, there is clearly some cross-over of these pathophysiological factors, which is an argument against considering NEC as truly separate diseases. In essence, NEC in term infants is not related to the risk factors peculiar to preterm infants but the corollary is that the risk factors for NEC in term infants are also associated with an increased risk in preterm babies.

In the following sections, multiple other aspects of NEC pathophysiology are explored. In each case there is both evidence and good mechanistic reasons to think that prematurity is an additive or synergistic factor in the pathogenesis of NEC. This helps us to build a fuller picture of the pathophysiology which is consistent with the observable fact that NEC is much more prevalent in premature babies but can still occur in those born at term.

5.3   Enteral Feeding

NEC is very rare in babies who have never been fed [16]. It is well-established that the risk of NEC is higher in babies who have received cows'-milk-based formula rather than breast milk. Therefore, it follows that enteral feeding is important to the pathogenesis of NEC. Conversely, given that NEC is primarily a disease of prematurity and is rarely seen in term infants in the absence of other known risk factors [17], it is arguably more correct to say that enteral feeding when the gut is not fully developed (or at risk because of other factors) is central to understanding how NEC develops.

The previous section covered some of the ways in which the premature intestine is not fully mature. This section will consider how adding in milk feeds to the intestine—which ideally should be quiescent because the infant remains in-utero—leads to pathology. Firstly, the epidemiological data clearly implicates enteral feeding—and indeed the choice of enteral feeds—as a key risk factor for NEC.

5.3.1   Breast Milk Versus Formula Milk

The risk of NEC is much higher in infants fed with cows' milk-based formula compared to those given maternal breast milk (MBM). Sisk et al. (2007) reported a sixfold reduction in the risk of NEC in infants fed on at least 50% maternal milk [18]. Furthermore, a dose effect of breast milk was found by Meinzen-Derr et al. (2009) in a secondary analysis of a cohort of 1272 infants [19]. In this study they found that the risk of the composite outcome of NEC or death was reduced with each 10% increase in the proportion of feed that was human milk.

5.3.2   Donor Breast Milk

If MBM is not available, donor breast milk (DBM) is an option for feeding neonates. Most developed countries have established 'milk-banks' and with many volunteer nursing mothers happy to provide milk. Indeed, in the UK, there is actually an excess of supply and it could be argued that neonatal units do not make as much use of this resource as they should. A Cochrane review of formula feeding versus donor breast milk for preterm infants had two important findings: Formula feed produced better growth trajectories but at the cost of a higher NEC risk [20, 21], These data suggest a nearly threefold increased risk of NEC in formula fed babies compared to DBM.

These two data sets suggest that the lowest risk of NEC for a preterm baby is milk from their own mother—followed by donor milk—followed by cows' milk-based formula. This begs a question as to why DBM would not be as protective as

MBM? The answer most likely lies in the way that DBM is handled prior to being given to a baby. The safety requirements for DBM in the UK means that it is pasteurised [22] which alters the protein and nutrient content. Specifically, it has been shown that DBM contains fewer immunoprotective factors than MBM [23]. Section 5.4 looks at the role of bacteria in causes NEC and Sect. 5.5 the role of the immune system. In summary though, DBM is not the same as MBM (due to the processing involved for safety reasons) and a demonstrable difference is seen with a reduction in immunoprotective factors which offers a very good explanation for the increased relative risk.

5.3.3 Enteral Nutrition and Growth in Preterm Babies

5.3.3.1 Neonatal Feed Fortifiers

There is an imperative to optimise nutrition in neonates as overall growth correlates with brain development. There is a clear association between poor growth in the neonatal period and poor neurodevelopmental outcomes [24] and there is some evidence that improving nutrition in the neonatal period reduces neurodevelopment impairment in preterm infants [25]. Unfortunately, human milk does not contain sufficient nutrients for a *pre-term* infant to grow. The compromise approach is to use breast milk feeds with fortifiers. However, that is not a risk-free option, either. The concern about fortifiers comes from anecdotal observations in clinical practice that babies often develop NEC whilst being given fortifiers. Historically, fortifiers were derived from non-human milk and hence there is a good rationale for expecting them to confer an NEC risk. An early trial was suggestive that there is indeed an increased risk with NEC rates of 5.8% compared with 2.2% in controls but this was not statistically significant [26]. However, a systematic review showed only limited evidence of an increased risk of NEC [27].

Currently, the European Society for Paediatric Gastroenterology Hepatology and Nutrition (ESPGHAN) guidelines recommend the use of human milk with nutrition fortifiers as 'standard practice [28].' This approach is designed to balance the need to reduce the risk of NEC with the need to support growth and development.

There are newer fortifier products now available which are based on human milk. Logically these may be the answer to how to have an exclusively human-milk fed baby and achieve sufficient calorific intake to support growth and development. However, they do come with a significant financial cost and studies do not currently exist to establish a clear benefit, to justify that cost.

5.3.3.2 Feed Volumes and Rate of Feeding Advancement

Logically, if feeding is a cause or trigger factor for NEC, then the amount of feed given, could be important. New born premature babies are started on low rates of milk feeds. These are then increased over the following days as tolerated. It was long thought that increasing the amount of feed relatively rapidly increased the risk or NEC. Indeed, historic observational studies tended to suggest that advancing feeds more rapidly was a trigger for NEC [29].

One randomised control trial of feed volumes had to be stopped early due to the number of babies who developed NEC in the 'progressive' group; [30] 141 infants were randomly assigned to a 'static' group or 'progressive group'.

In the static group, infants received 20 mL/kg/day of feeds for the first 10 days of life. The progressive group were given 20 mL/kg/day on day one, increasing by 20 mL/kg/day to a maximum of 140 mL/kg/day. The 'static' group had a rate of NEC of 1.4% compared to 10% in the 'progressive' group. This finding was not supported by subsequent studies and a Cochrane review concluded there was no benefit in advancing feeds more slowly. The ten studies included showed no difference in terms of the NEC risk between babies who advanced feeds 'rapidly' and those who's feed volumes were increased more slowly. It did show that delayed advancement in feeds lead to poorer growth with concerns about the potential impact on neurodevelopment in the long term [31, 32].

These studies do have limitations and so the Speed of Increasing Milk Feeds Trial (SIFT) was performed. The groups used for this study were a faster advancement group and a slower advancement group. The faster advancement group had their feeds increased by 30 mL per kg each day, whilst the slower group had their feeds increased by only 18 mL per kg per day. The results showed no difference in the NEC risk between the two groups (risk ratio 0.90 (95% CI 0.66 to 1.24)) [33]. The Cochrane review has since been updated and it remains the case that the best evidence we have at present is that the rate at which feeds are increased does not affect the risk of NEC.

5.3.4 Why Give Enteral Feeds at All?

NEC is very rare in babies who have not been fed. NEC is much more common in babies receiving formula milk compared to human milk. Therefore NEC is to some extent caused by enteral feeding.

In routine clinical practice it is relatively easy to provide nutrition without given anything enterally. There is the option of parenteral (intravenous) nutrition (PN). Theoretically, It would make sense to pursue a strategy of not giving enteral feeds at all in the first few weeks of life to babies born prematurely, in order to avoid this risk. However, this in itself carries significant risks and negative sequelae.

Delayed enteral feeding leads to higher rates of bloodstream infections and delayed gut development [15]. Indeed, animal models suggest that even delaying feeding for only a few days, leads to gut villi atrophy [34].

Whilst parenteral nutrition is a key part of the care of premature neonates, providing adequate nutrition for optimal growth via the parenteral route is challenging [35] (especially in terms of energy and protein content of the feed). Modern PN is quite sophisticated in the way that nutrients, electrolytes and trace elements can be matched to a patient's requirements, yet there remains a risk of liver impairment and multiple other issues. Especially with prolonged use. Central catheter infections also may well have a deleterious effect on neurodevelopment. Ultimately, the overall negative effects of withholding enteral feeds and giving parenteral nutrition significantly outweigh the potential benefit of reducing the NEC risk [36].

5.3.5   Enteral Feeding and the Pathogenesis of NEC

As Sections 5.3.1 to 5.3.4 show, the epidemiological relationship between enteral feeds and NEC is well-established with clear evidence that feeding confers a risk of NEC and there is clear evidence that some feeds are higher risk than others. As with prematurity, the epidemiology is a starting point for understanding how NEC develops. Why does feeding the premature gut cause this disease? Why, especially, is there such a big difference in risk between breast milk and cows' milk-based formulars?

The mechanism by which feeding confers a risk of NEC is not entirely established, although the association with immaturity is clearly important.

As noted above, in utero, the intestine is essentially at-rest. When the intestine is fulfilling its biological function of absorbing feeds, there is a much higher metabolic demand. The obvious implication here is that theoretically in a baby born prematurely, the intestine is not well-adapted to adopting this function.

5.3.5.1 Feeding and Metabolic Demand

The relationship between enteral feeding and NEC is partly explained by the increase in metabolic demand of the gut due to digestion and absorption of nutrients [37–39]. Indeed, in healthy infants, blood flow in the superior mesenteric artery

(SMA) is increased in response to feeds. This increase is greater in response to formula feeds than human milk [37]. This tells us two things; firstly—as would be expected—digesting and absorbing nutrients increases the metabolic demand on the intestine, necessitating an increase in blood flow. Secondly that absorption of formula feeds creates a higher demand than absorbing human milk. An inability of the intestine to respond to this need (potentially because of prematurity or other factors) appears to be a key part of the pathogenesis of NEC [40]. The metabolic demand and the ability of the intestine to respond to it will be discussed further in Sect. 5.7.

5.3.5.2   Formula Feeds

Other factors that may be important include the incomplete digestion and absorption of carbohydrates which leads to bacterial overgrowth [41]. The relative lactase deficiency of the premature infant means that lactose may be converted to short chain fatty acids by bacterial fermentation in the colon [42]. Over production of short chain fatty acids can cause mucosal injury in experimental animals [43]. The osmolality of feeds has long been a cause for concern. Human milk has an osmolality of approximately 300 mOsm/kg. This can be increased to more than 400 mOsm/kg with the addition of nutritional fortifiers [44]. Formula feeds can have an even higher osmolality but a recent systematic review showed there is no evidence of an increase in NEC risk with high osmolality feeds [45]. Although very high osmolality may be associated with delayed gastric emptying.

The effect of formula feeds on mucosal immunity seems to be significant both in terms of the pro-inflammatory effects of formula feeds and the absence of the immunological benefits of breast milk [41, 46, 47]. This is discussed further in Sect. 5.5.1.

5.4   Bacterial Colonisation

Bacterial colonisation is necessary for the development of NEC but not on its own sufficient to cause the disease. Ballance et al. (1990) showed that bacterial overgrowth is a feature of NEC specimens, and this is not seen in other intestinal conditions that are due to ischaemia [48]. This pathological finding implies a role for bacterial but does not answer the question whether infection is the initiating event in the pathophysiology or a secondary process. NEC is not seen in utero when the intestine is sterile. It classically develops around 10–14 days post birth which coincides with some of the changes of colonisation as the microbiome develops [49].

5.4.1 Pneumotosis Intestinalis

The pathognomonic feature of NEC radiologically is pneumotosis intestinalis; gas in the bowel wall (Fig. 7.1). Engel et al. presenting in 1973 at The Society for Pediatric Research and The American Pediatric Society Specialty Sessions described work done to ascertain the nature of the gas in the intestinal wall. They took surgical samples from babies with NEC and found that the intramural gas in both the lumen and the intestinal wall was at least 30% Hydrogen [50]. This is an important finding as hydrogen is not a product of human metabolism; implying a clear role for bacteria in the pathophysiology. Interestingly they cultured bacteria from the same patients and found that they were not producing hydrogen until they added in milk or 50% glucose to the culture medium. These findings were particularly important at the time as they were early direct evidence of a bacterial cause for NEC. They also imply that NEC involves bacterial invasion into the intestinal wall.

5.4.2 Bacteriology of the Neonatal Intestine

A prospective study that collected bacteriological and clinical data on all neonates less than 36 weeks of post conception age admitted to a single centre, revealed that all patients were colonised with potentially pathogenic bacteria in the week before contracting NEC [51]. Importantly, 79% of controls also had potentially pathogenic bacteria in their stools. This suggests that bacterial colonisation is a prerequisite for developing NEC but not on its own sufficient.

When NEC emerged in neonatal units, it was an early observation that NEC could exist in clusters—with several cases in the same unit in a short space of time, which implies an infective cause. Studies have shown that it can be possible to isolate specific organisms in these clusters [52].

NEC is not associated with one specific organism but studies have shown an association with different bacteria and even viral and fungal infections have been implicated [53]. These are based on both culture and molecular techniques to identify potential pathogens. Several studies have isolated specific organisms that seem to play some role in causing NEC, these include the bacteria *Escherichia coli, Pseudomonas aeruginosa, Klebsiella, Clostridium,* as well as Rotavirus, Adenovirus, CMV and fungal organisms including *Candida* [54].

What can be considered as 'depth of infection' is important (i.e. whether the bacterial invasion was only in the mucosa, or had progressed to the submucosa, muscularis or serosa). Remon et al. [55] found that the depth of infection in resected specimens correlated with the extent and depth of necrosis and with the mortality risk.

5.4.3 Development of the Microbiome

In recent years, in several contexts, the examination of the intestinal microbiome has become an area of significant research interest. Human health is hugely affected and altered by the mixture and proportion of bacteria species within the intestine. The intestinal flora play an important role in bile acid metabolism for example. There are thought to be many other roles that as yet we have not fully explored. In terms of NEC, the easiest way to understand the role of the microbiome is that it provides competitive exclusion of potentially pathogenic bacteria. Whilst it may well be more complex than this in reality, it is a logical hypothesis and is supported by the fact that several studies have shown that the administration of pro-biotics reduces the risk of NEC. The use of probiotics is discussed further in Sect. 6.5 Detailed studies suggest that providing commensal bacteria to the preterm gut has multiple positive effects, including; strengthening of the intestinal barrier, improved peristalsis and by stimulating mucin production [56].

The normal microbiome of the neonate is simple but also diverse and fluid. It has been described as having four distinct phases as it becomes more like that seen in older children and adults [49]. Phase 1 (birth to 2 weeks): *Streptococci* and coliforms predominate; Phase 2: Gram positive and non-spore-forming anaerobes emerge. Phase 3 coincides with the change of diet to solid food. The relative paucity of anerobes during Phase 1 allows pathogenic bacteria to colonize the neonatal gut more easily. The temporal association with the change from Phase 1 to Phase 2 and the typical timing of the onset of NEC supports the idea that this is an important factor.

Again, it is worth emphasising that the preterm intestine is different from the term infant's and that bacterial colonisation is apparently abnormal. It is not correct to think about bacterial colonisation as a risk factor without taking into account the fact that these are infants with an immature intestine. There is a lot of evidence to suggest that intestinal immunology is particularly affected by immaturity. This is the subject of the next section. In summary though, *colonisation of the intestine by potentially pathogenic bacteria is necessary but not sufficient for the development of NEC.* NEC specimens are characterised by bacterial overgrowth but NEC is not purely a disease caused by infection, as the histological findings are distinctly different from what is found in bacterial gastroenteritis.

5.5 Immunology

As noted in the previous section, consideration of the microbiome of babies that develop NEC without recognising the context of the immature and underdeveloped intestine is overly simplistic and potentially misleading. This is even more true when examining the immunological mechanisms that are part of the pathogenesis of

NEC. The immature intestine has an immature immune system. The colonisation of the intestinal tract plays an important role in the development and education of the immune system. As we have seen, the colonisation of the immature intestine is abnormal (compared to the term infant). Similarly, the immature intestine does not have normal motility or physical barriers to infection. Nevertheless, there has been considerable research interest in recent years in the specific role of the immune system in NEC pathology.

Cho et al. (2016) argue that NEC results from a profoundly dysregulated inflammatory response as a common endpoint of the various precipitating factors [57]. From this perspective, NEC is primarily an immune disease. This section will examine the role of the immune system in the pathogenesis of NEC.

5.5.1   Toll-Like Receptors

Toll-like receptors are potentially an elegant explanation of the origins of NEC. Their role in the disease fits with the observed risks of prematurity, bacterial colonisation and formula feeding, providing a mechanistic understanding of how these things fit together to cause this disease.

Experimental work with animal models of NEC suggest that the Toll-like receptors (TLRs) play an important role here, especially TLR4 [58]. In one model of NEC, TLR4-knockout mice do not develop the disease, implying a key role in the pathogenesis [59].

The Toll gene encodes for a protein which is important embryologically for determining the ventral-dorsal access. Toll-like receptors have a very different function but were named as such due to the similarity in their protein structure. This family of proteins are a group of transmembrane receptors that are a key part of the innate immune system [60]. They enable the immune system to respond to pathogens whether or not the individual has been exposed to that specific pathogen. This is clearly in stark contrast to antibodies which bind to specific antigens from specific organisms.

TLRs are found on both haemopoetic cells (i.e. immune cells) and non-haemopoetic cell types including enterocytes. They function by binding to structurally conserved molecules derived from bacteria, viruses and other microorganisms—i.e. these receptors are able to recognise a potential pathogen as bacterial or viral regardless of the actual species [61]. This is because microorganism have highly conserved structural motifs which are known as pathogen-associated microbial patterns (PAMPs). Or, to put it more simply, multiple proteins from diverse bacterial and other micro-organism species have proteins—or sections of proteins—which are very similar and hence are recognised as 'foreign' by the mammalian immune system. PAMPs are critical to the innate immune system being able to recognise invading organisms [62].

Receptors that bind PAMPs are collectively known as pattern recognition receptors (PRRs) [60]. PRRs will bind PAMPs on microorganisms within the intestine. This binding causes the TLRs to dimerise and recruit myeloid differentiation factor 88 (MyD88), which triggers down-stream signalling of the nuclear factor kappa beta pathway (NF-κβ) [63].

NF-κβ is a transcription factor that triggers an inflammatory response, bringing effector cells to the site of injury/invasion. This activation of TLR4 has been shown to result in increased enterocyte apoptosis, reduced enterocyte proliferation and migration and ultimately, breakdown of the intestinal epithelium.

In summary, the TLRs trigger an inflammatory response to microorganisms within the intestine and there is good evidence that this pathway is important in the pathogenesis of NEC.

TLR4 expression levels are higher in the premature gut compared to term controls. This nicely ties in with the fact that NEC is a disease of prematurity. Put simply, TLR4 expression is higher in premature neonates and therefore the premature bowel is more likely to have inflammation triggered by the TLR4 pathway and thus making the premature intestine much more vulnerable to NEC [58, 60, 64].

In a similar way, the role of TLR4 fits with the fact that prematurity if a key risk factor, it is also consistent with the role of Gram-negative bacteria in NEC. Lipopolysaccharide (LPS) is a major surface molecule of Gram-negative bacteria and is a potent stimulator of the innate immune response; it is the archetypal PAMP molecule [65]. LPS is a potent activator of TLR4 [66] and it has been shown that this triggers the NF-κβ inflammatory cascade [67]. Therefore the importance of TLR4 in the pathogenesis of NEC is consistent with the association with Gram-negative bacteria such as *Escherichia coli, Pseudomonas aeruginosa and Klebsiella* as discussed in Sect. 5.4.

5.5.1.1 TLR4 and Breast Milk

The role of toll-like receptors as a central, key trigger for NEC also fits with the effect of breast milk on NEC risk. Mouse studies have shown that breast milk attenuates TLR4 signalling [46]. This reduced activation of the TLR4 pathway could (at-least in part) explain the protective effect of breast milk.

As discussed in Sect. 5.3, breast milk confers a lower risk of NEC compared to cows' milk-based formula feeds. It is challenging to untangle the various factors involved: Is it the presence of various factors in formula that are not found in human milk that increase risk or does breast milk contain protective factors? Cumulative evidence would support both hypotheses. Recent work has shown that maternal Immunoglobulin A (IgA) is important in making this protective effect conferred by breast milk. Analysis of faecal cultures showed a decrease in IgA-bound bacteria preceding the onset on NEC in preterm babies [47]. Moreover in a mouse model of NEC, maternal milk is protective but this protective effect is abolished in IgA-deficient mothers. The importance of maternal IgA here seems to be in shaping the development of the neonatal microbiota and the absence of IgA in the gut allows the predominance of potentially pathogenic bacteria described in Sect. 5.4.3 to develop.

5.5.1.2 Toll-Like Receptors and NEC

It would be misleading to state that TLRs are the complete answer to the question of how NEC begins but it is very appealing as a key factor for the following reasons:

1. Experimental evidence shows it to be important in NEC
2. It triggers the NF-Kβ pathway which is known to be part of the pathogenesis
3. TLRs are a mechanism by which known risk factors can lead to NEC: They are over-expressed in the premature intestine; they respond to pathogens that are associated with NEC; and TLR-related inflammation is suppressed by breast milk.

5.5.2 Platelet Activating Factor

Another inflammatory mediator that has been implicated in the pathophysiology of NEC is Platelet activating factor (PAF). PAF is so-named because it was first identified as it causes platelets aggregation. Now it is known as a potent activator of inflammation.

In human studies, plasma levels of PAF have been shown to be higher in infants with NEC than healthy controls [68].

PAF is found in multiple tissues. Activation of PAF leads to epithelial cell damage and apoptosis. It affects leukocyte activation, platelet aggregation, cellular tight junctions and vasoconstriction [56]. PAF degradation is carried out by the enzyme PAF-acetylhydrolase (PAF-AH). In a rat model, PAF infusion leads to ischaemic bowel necrosis [69]. This intestinal injury can be prevented if the animals are pre-treated with medroxyprogesterone and dexamethasone which increase PAF-AH levels [70]. In short, PAF alone can induce an intestinal injury in animals that is analogous to NEC. Furthermore, the use of a PAF-antagonist significantly reduced the incidence of NEC In neonatal rats [71, 72]. Similarly, in a mouse model, PAF-AH knockout mice were far more susceptible to disease. This may be of just academic interest but maternal breast milk has detectable levels of PAF-AH [73]. PAF induction of TLR4 expression in the intestine has been demonstrated with quantitative PCR studies [74]. The importance of PAF in the human disease is difficult to ascertain. Arguably the interest in PAF is derived from the fact that its ability to produce a similar intestinal injury to NEC in animal models made it appealing as a means to studying the disease. Conversely the presence of PAF-AH in breast milk is an intriguing finding. Moreover, PAF triggering TLR-4 is consistent with the evidence for the key role of TLR-4 in NEC pathogenesis. However, it is probably too simplistic to tie the clinical observation that infants with NEC get thrombocytopenia to the role of PAF.

5.5.3 Neutrophils

The role of neutrophils in NEC pathophysiology remains unclear. In one animal study, neutrophils were depleted with vinblastine prior to inducing disease, which resulted in a reduced bowel necrosis [75]. Conversely, work in a different animal model showed that neutrophil depletion resulted in an increase in pro-inflammatory cytokines and enterocyte apoptosis [76]. So whilst the role of neutrophils specifically is perhaps enigmatic, these studies do both suggest that if neutrophils are playing a role it is by means of mediating inflammation rather than phagocytosis.

Moving from the animal to human studies, in infants that were small for gestational age, neutropenia was associated with an increased risk of developing NEC [77]. Neutrophils are a key part of the innate immune system, thus it is not surprising that they seem to be important in NEC but these conflicting data suggest that they may be both protective and play a role in promoting intestinal injury [60].

As such the exact role(s) of neutrophils are not well-understood. However it is known that PAF activates neutrophils, [78] so given the evidence of a potential role for PAF it would be logical that neutrophils do play a role in the pathophysiology of NEC and it might be that the effect of PAF is unrelated to platelets and is mediated by neutrophils or, indeed, by several other pathways.

5.5.4 Macrophages

The potential role of macrophages in the pathogenesis of NEC is another example of a mechanistic explanation as to why the risk of NEC is inversely related to gestational age.

Macrophages are best known for their role in phagocytosis of invading organisms. Indeed, intestinal macrophages are indeed very potent phagocytes [79]. However, they have multiple other functions: macrophages are important signalling cells that recruit and affect other immune cells. This role as important producers of a range of cytokines, necessary for an effective immune response, is important in NEC. This role as signalling cells is the subject of a lot of study and is quite complex but in simplistic terms, one can consider macrophages to be pro-inflammatory or anti-inflammatory.

Detailed analysis of intestinal macrophages suggests that pro-inflammatory macrophages are a different sub-population from the resident macrophages that have a phagocytic activity against invading organisms [80]. Resident intestinal macrophages are profoundly inactive in terms of producing an inflammatory response in normal circumstances [81]. They phagocytose organisms without stimulating inflammation.

Macrophage-rich infiltrates in both the inflamed and non-inflamed mucosa are found in NEC [55, 82] and these macrophages contrast with the normal intestinal macrophage in that they have a pro-inflammatory profile [83]. Tumour growth factor beta (TGF-β) suppresses the inflammatory profile of macrophages. Maheshwari et al. showed that intestinal macrophages acquire a non-inflammatory profile during maturation of the premature gut. This maturation is mediated by the expression of TGF-β [84]. Subsequently, MohanKumar et al. demonstrated that expression of Smad7 (SMAD family member 7) in response to bacterial products interrupts the TGF-β -mediated inflammatory downregulation of macrophages and promotes NF-κβ activation [83].

Taken together these findings provide a pathway by which bacteria induce a profound inflammatory response that is seen in NEC and provide some explanation as to why premature babies would be at greater risk. The premature intestine, if the infant remained in-utero, would remain sterile and the macrophages would not be exposed to antigens. With premature birth, the intestine is colonised at an earlier stage of its normal maturation. Hence, the macrophages are exposed to bacteria and the normal maturation to being anti-inflammatory cells (mediated by TGF-β) is interrupted. Therefore the intestine is more prone to inflammation and therefore at increased risk of developing NEC.

5.5.5 Lymphocytes

T-lymphocytes are known to be important in the development of NEC [60]. T-lymphocytes are characterised by the presence of a T-cell receptor (TCR) which binds to antigens. In adults (and older children), the majority of T-lymphocytes are referred to as αβ T-cells because the TCR is made up of these two subunits. There is another, much smaller population of T-lymphocytes with different subunits making up the TCR, these are known as γδ T-cells as the receptor is formed of two different but analogous subunits—γ and δ. In the premature neonate the γδ T-cells in the intestine are far more active and produce higher levels of cytokines including IFN-γ and IL-10 [85].

Weitkamp et al. found that these γδ lymphocytes are depleted in infants that contracted NEC compared to controls [86]. Thus, we have two intriguing findings with the T-cell population; namely that γδ cell are much more populous in the preterm neonatal gut and that the population of T-cells changes in NEC. This is very good evidence that they are important in the pathogenesis of NEC but the exact role is less clear. The higher level of γδ cells may be pro-inflammatory which is similar to the pattern seen with macrophages—the premature intestine is more prone to inflammation than the gut of a term infant. The drop in this population of cells associated with NEC is not so easily explained. Is it a cause or effect of NEC? One clue that may help us untangle this is that γδ cells are thought to be critical in maintaining barrier integrity [60] but it does remains an intriguing question.

Regulatory T-cells primary function is to suppress the immune response and thus their dysfunction is associated with inflammation. In human NEC specimens, populations of regulatory cells are reduced [86]. Conversely, CD-17+ T-helper cells (a recognised subgroup of T-helper cells) produce a range of cytokines that cause intestinal inflammation. Egan et al. demonstrated in a mouse model that regulatory T-cells are reduced whilst these pro-inflammatory CD17+ T-helper cells are increased [87]. These T-cells produce high levels of IL-17A that results in a loss of tight-junctions between epithelial cells, reduced enterocyte proliferation and increased apoptosis in intestinal crypts. Moreover they found that TLR-4 caused the influx of these CD17+ lymphocytes.

T-cell populations and functions are clearly altered in NEC. It would be an overstatement to say that the mechanism is fully understood but in simple terms, there is a lot of evidence that there is immune dysregulation which is inherently pro-inflammation that leads to the development of NEC.

5.5.6 Genetic Factors

As noted in Chap. 4, the incidence of NEC varies considerably between different populations. For example, NEC is less common in Austria, Japan and Switzerland and more common in the UK, Ireland, and North America [88]. Implicitly, there are multiple potential explanations for these differences. It could be attributed to differences in neonatal care, for example. However studies limited to neonatal units only in the USA demonstrated that there were differences linked to race alone. African-American infants are at greater risk of NEC than Caucasians [89, 90] Furthermore, twin studies have demonstrated significant concordance [91].

NEC is undoubtedly an acquired rather than congenital condition but there could be multiple genetic factors that may predispose an infant to NEC. As discussed above (Sect. 5.5.1), TLR4 appears to be very important in the triggering of the inflammatory pathways which lead to NEC. Therefore it is logical to hypothesise TLR4 polymorphisms might confer risk but thus far no such predisposing alleles have (as yet) been identified [92]. Similarly, research into genetic variations of pro-inflammatory cytokines, the NF-κ β pathway and PAF have yet to yield conclusive results [92].

At the time of writing, there exists epidemiological evidence that genetic factors do exist that will predispose an infant to NEC. There are several candidate genes and pathways in the immune system that would explain this predisposition but as yet there is no direct evidence for any specific genes conferring an increased risk.

5.6   Ischaemia-Reperfusion Injury

Ischaemia-reperfusion injury (IRI) occurs in severe different pathologies, including coronary heart disease and stroke. IRI involves a loss of an adequate blood supply for a period of time (ischaemia), followed by the restoration of the blood supply (reperfusion) which results in significant tissue or organ damage [93]. The loss of an adequate blood supply is implicitly a non-sustainable state for a prolonged period of time. The paradox is that with short periods of ischaemia (such that the tissue survives), the majority of the damage is done during the reperfusion phase [94]. The concept of an adequate blood supply is critical here as how much perfusion is required at any given time is related to the work the organ or tissue is doing and therefore its metabolic demand. The archetypal example of this is stable angina. At rest, with the cardiac tissue doing relatively little work, the patient has no symptoms. However with exercise, the metabolic demand of the cardiac muscle increases and thus the amount of blood flow in the coronary arteries required also increases. Stable angina is the result of coronary vessel disease meaning that the needed increase in flow is not possible.

It is analogous to the intestine in as much as the metabolic demand of intestinal tissue also varies significantly. In normal health the intestinal capillary blood flow needs to increase in response to the need to absorb feed (or indeed in response to inflammation).

5.6.1   Evidence That Demonstrates Ischaemia-Reperfusion Injury Is Part of Necrotising Enterocolitis

There remains some debate about the role of IRI in the pathogenesis of NEC. Some early papers suggested that NEC was primarily an IRI disease. More recently, there has been more focus on the role of inflammation and immune dysregulation. Ultimately though, the histological picture of NEC is ischaemic necrosis [48]. Whatever else is going on in this disease, IRI is the end point that is seen in surgical specimens.

The seminal paper on NEC histology is Ballance et al. (1990) [48]. This was a series of intestinal surgical or autopsy specimens from 84 patients with NEC. In this series, 89% had ischaemic necrosis. In the discussion they wrote *"The histological picture of NEC is inescapably similar to that of other bowel diseases known to be ischaemic in origin."* The also noted that the bacterial overgrowth seen in NEC is not a feature of other ischaemic diseases but *"...the pathological changes of NEC are distinctly different from those of infective enteritis or colitis in older patients."* One other important finding in this series is that the majority of specimens showed reparative changes in the intestine which means that NEC is not a single 'hit' on this intestine but a disease that progresses over hours or days.

Whilst NEC can be found in any area of the intestine, it is most commonly seen in the terminal ileum which is consistent with an ischaemic process as this area is supplied by vessels which are more distal from the superior mesenteric artery than other parts of the bowel.

NEC in term babies is associated primarily with congenital cardiac disease—more specifically with low cardiac-output states. Studies of risk-factors for NEC in term infants have identified several factors associated with an increased risk which include polycythaemia, sepsis and hypotension (see Table 4.4). Each of these could credibly be linked to NEC by IRI by the fact that they result in relatively poor perfusion of the gut. A recent Cochrane review on oxygen therapy in neonates demonstrated that targeting lower oxygen saturation levels in premature neonates (to reduce the risk of retinopathy) resulted in higher rates of NEC [95].

Historically, it was proposed that the so-called 'diving reflex' may be the explanation for these findings [96]. The diving reflex is a very primitive reflex that diverts blood flow away from the intestine to vital organs. This reflex, which allows sustained perfusion to the brain and heart, but ultimately results in intestinal injury [97], was thought to be induced by various stresses in the perinatal period. More recently, the evidence has very much undermined that theory with much more focus on the immunological and microbiological aspects [98].

It is certainly incorrect to think of NEC as a purely ischaemic disease [98] akin to coronary vessel disease or stroke, but the histopathology of NEC is one of ischaemic necrosis so the real question is one of the sequence of causative factors. In the simplest terms, IRI is the common end pathway of the factors discussed previously.

More recently, we have more direct evidence of an ischaemic process in NEC. Chen et al. (2016) [99] investigated the ischaemic markers hypoxia-inducible factor-1 (HIF-1) and glucose transporter 1 (Glut1) in histological specimens of patients with NEC who underwent surgical resection.

HIF-1 is a transcription factor made of two subunits (HIF-1α and HIF-1β) and is a key part of the cell's response to hypoxia. Hence it is a marker of hypoxic insult at the cellular level. Neither HIF-1α or HIF-1β have any known function independently but the combination of the two subunits to form HIF-1 results in altered gene expression downstream. Under normoxic conditions HIF-1α has very high turnover. It is constitutively expressed and very rapidly broken down by proteasomal degradation. The function of the enzyme responsible for this breakdown is oxygen dependent and therefore hypoxia inhibits the breakdown of HIF-1α, leading to its nuclear accumulation and a functioning HIF-1 molecule [100]. The HIF-1 molecule, acting as a transcription factor activates multiple genes, including Glut-1. Chen et al. used tissue from patients with small bowel volvulus or resection from an incarcerated hernia to confirm that both HIF-1α and Glut-1 are expressed in the epithelial layer of bowel exposed to ischaemia. Having confirming the role of HIF-1α and Glut-1 as a reliable marker in neonatal gut tissue, they studied bowel specimens from patients with severe NEC. These specimens had the same 'ischaemic-type' pattern of HIF-1α and Glut-1 expression [99].

5.6.2   Gut Immaturity and Ischaemia-Reperfusion Injury

The intestine of the adult or term neonate regulates its blood flow allowing a significant increase in flow in response to the increased metabolic demand of feeding (or inflammation). The immature bowel is not able to regulate its blood flow in the same way and hence, if the intestine is absorbing feed or undergoing inflammation there will be relative ischaemia at the mucosal level.

As discussed in Sect. 5.3.5, there is a strong imperative to give enteral feeds to neonates, even those born prematurely. This inevitably means an increased perfusion demand in the gut circulation [37–39]. In essence, the premature intestine is much less able to cope with the increased demand than the bowel of a term neonate.

The regulation of blood flow in the intestinal circulation is controlled by the antagonistic actions of endothelin-1 (ET-1) and nitric oxide (NO) which regulate intestinal vascular resistance. ET-1 increases vascular resistance and therefore decreases flow, whilst NO causes localised vasodilation and increases flow. Any alteration of this balance towards ET-1, causes vasoconstriction and consequential intestinal ischaemia as the intestinal blood flow is reduced and there is insufficient perfusion to meet the metabolic demand [98].

There is good evidence from both animal and human studies to support this model of the intestinal circulation. Downard et al. (2011) used an animal model and showed that altered microcirculation is a critical event in the pathogenesis of NEC [40]. With real-time observation of the microvasculature, they observed arteriole diameters were significantly smaller in animals who developed NEC, compared to controls who did not. Similarly, it has been shown that there is a correlation between early tolerance of enteral feeds and an increase in blood flow velocity in the superior-mesenteric artery (SMA). High SMA resistance (which implies that inflow will be impaired) demonstrated on ultrasonography in human infants is a predictor of the development of NEC [101, 102].

The occurrence of NEC in term infants with congenital heart disease(CHD), especially low-output states, similarly supports the notion that under-perfusion is a trigger for NEC. Babies who suffer poor perfusion or shock are the ones who subsequently develop NEC [103]. In this context, it could be argued that NEC is simply an IRI disease with the subsequent bacterial infection of the bowel wall resulting when the initial ischaemic injury causing a break-down in the barrier function of the intestinal wall.

The unanswered question has always been that if IRI is the key here, why do preterm infants with normal vascular anatomy and no obvious global under-perfusion like the child with CHD, also suffer an ischaemia-reperfusion injury?

This can be explained by considering that the increased metabolic demand of feeding, the insult of infection and inflammation seen in preterm babies, especially those fed on formula—coupled with the immature gut's inability to regulate perfusion in response to metabolic demand - leads to mucosal ischaemia. This kind of synergistic relationship between tissue hypoxia and formula feeding has been demonstrated in a mouse model [104].

Implicitly, inflammation increases the blood flow requirement. Inflammation is a high flow state as fluid losses from micro vessels increase and the metabolic demand of inflammatory processes are higher than baseline. Hence inflammation implies a need for increased blood flow and if the immature intestine is unable to meet this need there will be localised ischaemia.

There is also a more specific link between the immunological pathways of NEC and ischaemia. The role of TLR4 discussed is part of this as TLR4 impairs intestinal perfusion directly by inhibiting endothelial nitric oxide synthase (eNOS). eNOS synthase—as its name implies—synthesises NO in the endothelium which (as discussed above) is a key pathway for causing vasodilation in the intestinal microcirculation [105]. This reduction in microcirculation causes localised ischaemia [61]. The importance of eNOS has been further demonstrated by administration of sildenafil (a phosphodiesterase-5 inhibitor) to maintain intraluminal nitric oxide activity in a mouse model resulting in markedly reduced NEC severity. In contrast, eNOS-deficient mice have much greater disease severity [105]. As discussed in Sect. 5.5.1, TLR4 is expressed at a higher level in the preterm intestine, compared to full-term controls [61]. Here we see a direct link between the predilection towards TLR-mediated inflammation in the immature intestine and the end-point of ischaemic necrosis [48].

This understanding of NEC with IRI at the mucosal level as a common pathway from multiple factors, is further supported by the fact that systemic factors (such as hypoxia) increase the risk of NEC [95].

5.6.3   *Ischaemia-Reperfusion Injury and NEC Risk-Factors*

As previously noted, NEC is virtually never seen in term neonates without specific risk factors [17] and the same risk factors increase the risk of NEC in premature infants as well [15]. This is part of the evidence base that supports the notion that NEC in term neonates and 'classical' NEC in preterm babies is part of the same disease entity or at least there is significant commonality between the disease in term babies and pre-term. Although, it must be noted that there is clearly significant heterogeneity in NEC.

This variation does lead some to argue that NEC should be considered as multiple disease entities [106]. Whilst this may well be a correct approach, this overlap in risk-factors between term and preterm infants strongly suggests some sort of common pathway as well.

5.6.4 Congenital Cardiac Disease and NEC Risk

NEC is a disease of prematurity. As has been noted, that does not mean that NEC does not occur in term neonates. The 10% of cases that occur in term babies represents a significant minority. Most of these cases will be babies with congenital heart disease (CHD) [107].

It is possible that there is an embryological or genetic explanation for this increased risk. There could be a common causative factor for both CHD and NEC but a more straight-forward explanation is that poor intestinal perfusion and thus intestinal IRI is the key pathogenic step in this group who develop NEC. This hypothesis is further supported by the fact that NEC is seen most commonly in the infants with CHD that have a low-output state and poor systemic perfusion [108].

Unlike NEC seen in preterm infants, the most common site of bowel injury in CHD babies is the colon [107] (in contrast to the terminal ileum in 'classical' NEC.) although there is no clear explanation for why the colon should be more susceptible in this group.

Again, the association between CHD and NEC is indicative of the role IRI plays in NEC.

5.6.5 Intrauterine Growth Restriction (IUGR)

There are multiple neonatal risks associated with in-utero factors such as maternal pre-eclampsia and intrauterine growth restriction (IUGR) [109]. Factors that impact development in-utero continue to have effects on the neonate after birth.

In late pregnancy, with the placenta providing equivalent function to the lungs, the intestine and the kidneys, it is unsurprising that it requires a significant proportion of cardiac output. In the second trimester, a third of the foetal cardiac output will go to the placenta. In IUGR this fraction is reduced, in extreme cases to one-tenth [110].

During antenatal scans, foetal Doppler assessment of the umbilical arteries can detect absent or reversed end-diastolic flow (AREDF) velocity which corresponds to this extreme under perfusion. A 2010 Cochrane review recommended the use of Doppler ultrasound in high risk pregnancies. This was subsequently withdrawn, pending further evidence and an update [111].

The presence of AREDF has been associated with a higher risk of NEC [112]. The mechanism here is not simple. The concept that intestinal perfusion is reduced to preferentially support circulation to the brain, heart and kidneys is well established [110]. Why this in-utero insult impacts on intestinal risk of NEC weeks later is not fully understood. Several mechanisms could be proposed such as the relative under perfusion of the intestine delaying gut development and maturity.

This increased risk led to the logical hypothesis that delaying feeds in infants that had been identified as being high-risk antenatally would be a wise precaution to reduce the NEC risk. However, a trial of early versus late feeding in infants with AREDF showed that delaying feeds did not reduce the risk of NEC but did increase the need for parenteral nutrition [113].

Whether AREDF fits with an IRI mechanism in NEC is also not clear. Strictly speaking, the relative under perfusion of the intestine in-utero due to AREDF is not an ischaemic hit in the right timeframe to be a causative factor for NEC. However, if the under perfusion persists into ex-utero life then it would make the intestine more vulnerable to NEC. There is no clear evidence for this so it is an open question as to whether this is relates to how IRI is part of NEC pathophysiology.

5.6.6 Transfusion-Associated Necrotising Enterocolitis and Anaemia

The association between red blood cell (RBC) transfusions and NEC has been the subject of study for some time. The causative relationship between RBC transfusions and NEC has been considered strong enough that the term *TANEC* (transfusion-associated necrotising enterocolitis) [114] was coined.

A potential mechanism that has been proposed is that RBC transfusion could cause a TRALI-like (transfusion-related lung injury-like) reaction in the intestine which would cause intestinal inflammation, leading to NEC [115].

Whilst there exists a rationale for thinking that RBC transfusion can trigger NEC, the best evidence available suggests that transfusion is more likely to be a confounder and that anaemia is the risk factor for NEC rather than the blood transfusion.

A 2019 trial by Janjindamai et al. included over 400 very low birth weight (VLBW) infants. This trial with babies at the highest risk of NEC showed no association with RBC transfusions and NEC after controlling for confounders [116]. Similarly, Hay et al.'s previous review found that when the GRADE (Grading of recommendations assessment, development and evaluation) system was applied to the literature on TANEC, the overall quality of the evidence that RBC transfusion conferred a risk of NEC was 'very low' [114].

One of the great problems with all the studies in this area is that it is very difficult to avoid confounders. The most obvious—and most important—confounder here is anaemia. An observational study by Patel et al. reported that severe anaemia (defined as a haemoglobin level of less than 8 g/dL) is associated with a sixfold increase in NEC risk in the following week. This increase was independent of whether the patients received a transfusion [117]. Although, it should be noted that the reported cause-specific hazard ratio (HR) of 5.99 had a very wide 95% confidence interval (2.00–18.0). Importantly, additional analysis showed a dose effect. With each 1 g/dL decrease in the nadir of haemoglobin they found a 65% increase in the risk of NEC. These data are strong evidence for the notion that anaemia rather than RBC transfusion is the more likely risk factor for NEC. This does not exclude reverse-causation, however.

It many neonatal units, it is standard practice to withhold feeding whilst transfusions are being given. This is a logical step to reduce the stress on this intestine whilst the transfusion is running. Despite this being routine practice, several studies have shown no increased risk with continuing feeding whilst giving RBC transfusions [118], again reinforcing support for the argument that anaemia rather than transfusion is the actual risk for NEC.

As noted, transfusion could plausibly cause or augment injury to the intestine but the same is also true of anaemia. Anaemia is known to impair splanchnic perfusion resulting in tissue hypoxia and anaerobic metabolism [119]. If anaemia is indeed the true association with NEC (rather than RBC transfusion) that lends further support for the concept of NEC as an IRI disease. Tissue hypoxia, secondary to anaemia leads to or increases intestinal injury. Anaemia is significant for the development of NEC in that global anaemia will lead to (relative) intestinal hypoxia.

Conversely, it there is an inflammatory reaction in the intestine from transfusion that in itself would increase the metabolic demand of the tissue causing relative ischaemia. Therefore if RBC transfusion is the culprit, it does not exclude an IRI explanation for NEC whilst the clearer association with anaemia is strong evidence that IRI is important for the development of NEC.

5.6.7   Patent Ductus Arteriosus

The foetal circulation is distinctly different from adult circulation as it allows the majority of oxygenated blood from the placenta to bypass the lungs and enter the systemic circulation. In utero, the ductus arteriosus along with the foramen ovale allows this bypass to occur. The foramen ovale begins to close when an infant takes its first breath and in a term infant, the duct will normally close within 72 h of birth [120].

Failure of this closure and hence a *patent ductus arteriosus* (PDA) (beyond 72 h) occurs in the majority of preterm infants. PDA is reported at over 70% in babies born before 28 weeks [121] and 80% in those born between 24 and 25 weeks gesation [122].

After birth, a PDA usually results in a left-to-right (systemic to pulmonary) shunt due to the pressure difference between the systemic and pulmonary circulations. The presence of a shunt is not necessarily of any clinical significance and a shunt only really matters if it has a meaningful haemodynamic effect. Unfortunately, there is very little consensus as what constitutes a haemodynamically significant PDA (hsPDA) [120]. It has been shown that a hsPDA (by whichever definition) results in lower splanchnic oxygenation [123] and therefore plausabily a hsPDA would be expected to increase the risk of NEC. A hsPDA is simply another mechanism by which the intestine would be relatively under perfused.

However, there is no direct evidence of an increased risk from a PDA. Partly this is due to the fact that PDAs are extremely common in preterm neonates. Demonstrating that a PDA is an independent risk-factor for NEC is challenging because of the near-ubiquity of PDAs in preterm infants: The majority of the at-risk population will have one [121, 122]. Recent data shows no clear link between hsPDA and developing NEC [124]. Studies designed to look at the benefit of treating PDAs have shown no benefit in terms of reduced mortality from treating even a haemodynamically significant PDA [125].

In contrast there is some evidence that treating a PDA can reduce the risk of NEC as a detailed review and meta-analysis of PDA treatments did show that high-dose ibuprofen treatment did reduce the risk of developing NEC [126].

Whilst this is clearly not a strong evidence base it further builds up our picture of how haemodynamic factors effect NEC risk. The left to right shunt of a PDA leads to reduce oxygenation of the intestine. This is again support for an IRI mechanism being important in the pathology of NEC.

5.6.8   Ischaemia-Reperfusion Injury as a Common End-Pathway for Necrotising Enterocolitis Pathophysiology

Throughout this chapter, several predisposing factors that have been implicated in NEC have been reviewed. The role of immune dysregulation is undoubtedly important in NEC but IRI is inescapably part of the pathogenesis. This is clear because of the histological findings. Whatever else is happening with NEC, ischaemic necrosis is what a pathologist finds in surgical or autopsy specimens.

Especially in the term infant [17], but also in the pre-term infant [15] there are a group of risk factors (i.e. sepsis, polycythaemia and hypotension) that result in compromised bowel perfusion. In the term infant, NEC is virtually never seen without one or more of these risk factors. In preterm babies, the risk of NEC is demonstrably higher in the presence of these risk factors.

IRI as a pathological feature of NEC fits with each of these risk factors: mild systemic hypoxia may be well tolerated by the intestine. Similarly, the increased metabolic demand of absorbing feeds may, on its own not result in intestinal injury. Inflammation triggered by bacterial overgrowth may result in only minimal injury. However when one or more of these factors is combined, it is highly likely to result in a localised IRI resulting in tissue necrosis. IRI itself triggers a pronounced inflammatory response [127]. Compromise of the bowel wall enables bacterial invasion, a cardinal sign of NEC [48, 50].

This understanding makes IRI a secondary event rather than the primary cause [106, 128]. However, it is arguably more accurate to describe this as a vicious cycle as IRI triggers further inflammation [129] and necrosis is a major driver of inflammation leading to further ischaemia [130]. Similarly, localised injury resulting in compromise of the bowel wall enables bacterial invasion whilst bacterial invasion of the intestinal wall will cause inflammation.

This is consistent with the clinical and histological evidence that NEC is an evolving disease process rather than a singular event [48].

5.7 A Coherent Understanding?

A complete understanding of NEC pathophysiology must incorporate all the risk factors discussed here as the epidemiological evidence for each of them is very strong. How to tie this together with the other evidence that we have about the mechanisms involved in the pathophysiology is the purpose of this chapter. Undoubtedly, NEC is a disease that occurs predominately in premature neonates. Undoubtedly NEC is related to feeds. Similarly, we have good evidence that there is immune dysfunction resulting in inflammation and that there is an ischaemia-reperfusion injury to the intestine. It is also the case that bacterial infection is a necessary component of the disease process.

It is a mistake to think of NEC as a one-time event. As noted, there are reparative changes and NEC is a disease that develops over several hours to a few days. It is also a mistake to think about any of the causative factors in isolation—clearly there is significant synergy between them. And finally it is a mistake to think of NEC as a chain of events. It is a cycle whereby inflammation causes further compromise and increases the risk of further damage. Injury to the intestinal wall, facilitates bacterial invasion, triggering inflammation and inflammation causes damage to the intestinal wall leading to bacterial invasion. All of these processes increase the metabolic demand in the intestine to which (in the pre-term neonate especially) it is not able to adapt, leading to ischaemia of the tissue.

Figure 5.1 is a schematic that brings all these factors together. The green boxes represent known risk factors for NEC. The red and blue boxes represent pathways that have been shown by empirical evidence to be involved in how NEC starts and progresses and the red boxes are common end pathways. The most important aspect of this is the multiple direction of the arrows, emphasising the vicious cycle that occurs in NEC pathogenesis.

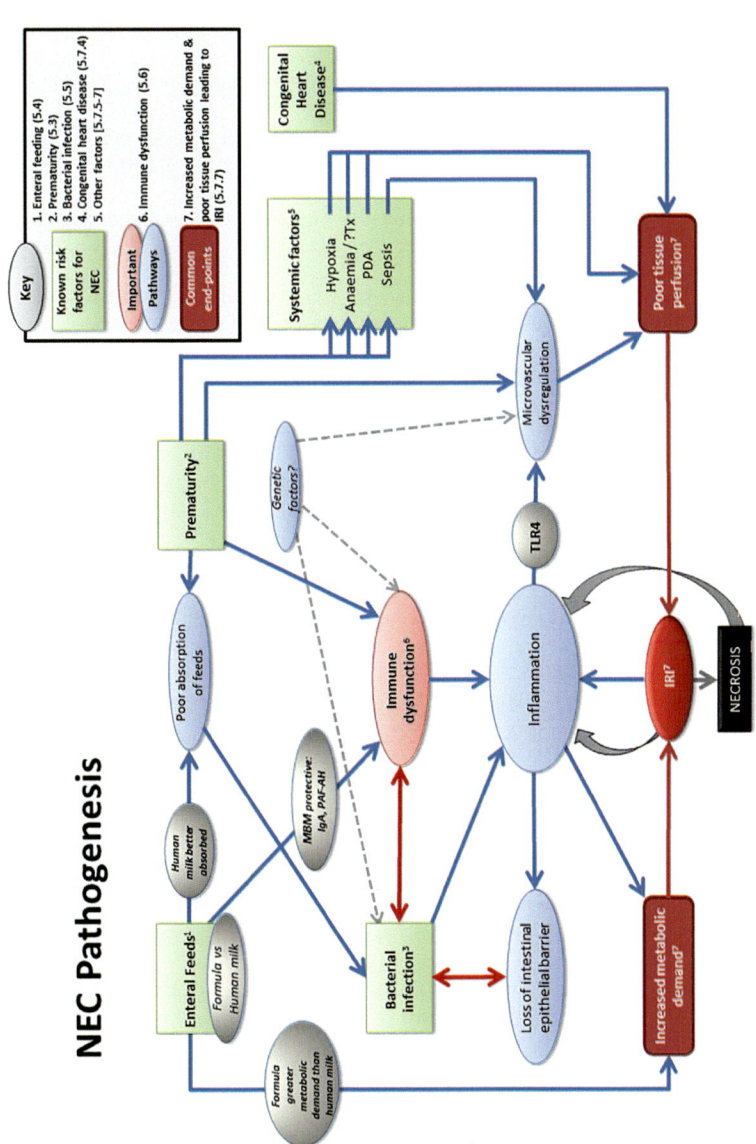

Fig. 5.1 NEC pathophysiology

References

1. Lin PW, Stoll BJ. Necrotising enterocolitis. Lancet. 2006;368(9543):1271–83. https://doi. org/10.1016/s0140-6736(06)69525-1.
2. Lebenthal A, Lebenthal E. The ontogeny of the small intestinal epithelium. JPEN J Parenter Enteral Nutr. 1999;23(5 Suppl):S3–6. https://doi.org/10.1177/014860719902300502.
3. Fitzgibbons SC, Ching Y, Yu D, Carpenter J, Kenny M, Weldon C, et al. Mortality of necrotizing enterocolitis expressed by birth weight categories. J Pediatr Surg. 2009;44(6):1072–5.; ; discussion 5–6. https://doi.org/10.1016/j.jpedsurg.2009.02.013.
4. Luig M, Lui K. Epidemiology of necrotizing enterocolitis—part II: risks and susceptibility of premature infants during the surfactant era: a regional study. J Paediatr Child Health. 2005;41(4):174–9. https://doi.org/10.1111/j.1440-1754.2005.00583.x.
5. Yee WH, Soraisham AS, Shah VS, Aziz K, Yoon W, Lee SK. Incidence and timing of presentation of necrotizing enterocolitis in preterm infants. Pediatrics. 2012;129(2):e298–304. https://doi.org/10.1542/peds.2011-2022.
6. Berseth CL. Gastrointestinal motility in the neonate. Clin Perinatol. 1996;23(2):179–90.
7. Dinsmore JE, Jackson RJ, Smith SD. The protective role of gastric acidity in neonatal bacterial translocation. J Pediatr Surg. 1997;32(7):1014–6.
8. Hyman PE, Clarke DD, Everett SL, Sonne B, Stewart D, Harada T, et al. Gastric acid secretory function in preterm infants. J Pediatr. 1985;106(3):467–71.
9. Lebenthal E, Lee PC. Development of functional responses in human exocrine pancreas. Pediatrics. 1980;66(4):556–60.
10. Buisine MP, Devisme L, Savidge TC, Gespach C, Gosselin B, Porchet N, Aubert JP. Mucin gene expression in human embryonic and fetal intestine. Gut. 1998;43(4):519–24.
11. Eckmann L. Innate immunity and mucosal bacterial interactions in the intestine. Curr Opin Gastroenterol. 2004;20(2):82–8.
12. Mallow EB, Harris A, Salzman N, Russell JP, DeBerardinis RJ, Ruchelli E, Bevins CL. Human enteric defensins. Gene structure and developmental expression. J Biol Chem. 1996;271(8):4038–45.
13. Gallo R, Hooper L. Epithelial antimicrobial defence of the skin and intestine. Nat Rev Immunol. 2012;12(7):503–16. https://doi.org/10.1038/nri3228.
14. Neu J. Necrotizing enterocolitis. Semin Fetal Neonatal Med. 2018;23(6):369. https://doi. org/10.1016/j.siny.2018.08.009.
15. Gephart SM, McGrath JM, Effken JA, Halpern MD. Necrotizing enterocolitis risk: state of the science. Adv Neonatal Care. 2012;12(2):77–87; quiz 8–9. https://doi.org/10.1097/ ANC.0b013e31824cee94.
16. Berseth CL. Feeding strategies and necrotizing enterocolitis. Curr Opin Pediatr. 2005;17(2):170–3.
17. Lambert DK, Christensen RD, Henry E, Besner GE, Baer VL, Wiedmeier SE, et al. Necrotizing enterocolitis in term neonates: data from a multihospital health-care system. J Perinatol. 2007;27(7):437–43. https://doi.org/10.1038/sj.jp.7211738.
18. Sisk P, Lovelady C, Dillard R, Gruber K, O'Shea T. Early human milk feeding is associated with a lower risk of necrotizing enterocolitis in very low birth weight infants. J Perinatol. 2007;27(7):428–33. https://doi.org/10.1038/sj.jp.7211758.
19. Meinzen-Derr J, Poindexter B, Wrage L, Morrow A, Stoll B, Donovan E. Role of human milk in extremely low birth weight infants' risk of necrotizing enterocolitis or death. J Perinatol. 2009;29(1):57–62. https://doi.org/10.1038/jp.2008.117.
20. Quigley MA, Henderson G, Anthony MY, McGuire W. Formula milk versus donor breast milk for feeding preterm or low birth weight infants. Cochrane Database Syst Rev. 2007;4:CD002971. https://doi.org/10.1002/14651858.CD002971.pub2.
21. Quigley M, McGuire W. Formula versus donor breast milk for feeding preterm or low birth weight infants. Cochrane Database Syst Rev. 2014;4:CD002971. https://doi. org/10.1002/14651858.CD002971.pub3.

22. National Institute for Health and Care Excellence. Donor milk banks: service operation. Clinical Guidance 2010 [Internet]. 2010. https://www.nice.org.uk/guidance/CG93. Accessed 11 Dec 2020.
23. Bertino E, Giuliani F, Baricco M, Di Nicola P, Peila C, Vassia C, et al. Benefits of donor milk in the feeding of preterm infants. Early Hum Dev. 2013;89(Suppl 2):S3–6. https://doi.org/10.1016/j.earlhumdev.2013.07.008.
24. Ehrenkranz R, Dusick A, Vohr B, Wright L, Wrage L, Poole W. Growth in the neonatal intensive care unit influences neurodevelopmental and growth outcomes of extremely low birth weight infants. Pediatrics. 2006;117(4):1253–61. https://doi.org/10.1542/peds.2005-1368.
25. Chan S, Johnson M, Leaf A, Vollmer B. Nutrition and neurodevelopmental outcomes in preterm infants: a systematic review. Acta Paediatr. 2016;105(6):587–99. https://doi.org/10.1111/apa.13344.
26. Lucas A, Fewtrell MS, Morley R, Lucas PJ, Baker BA, Lister G, Bishop NJ. Randomized outcome trial of human milk fortification and developmental outcome in preterm infants. Am J Clin Nutr. 1996;64(2):142–51.
27. Sullivan S, Schanler RJ, Kim JH, Patel AL, Trawoger R, Kiechl-Kohlendorfer U, et al. An exclusively human milk-based diet is associated with a lower rate of necrotizing enterocolitis than a diet of human milk and bovine milk-based products. J Pediatr. 2010;156(4):562–7.e1. https://doi.org/10.1016/j.jpeds.2009.10.040.
28. Agostoni C, Buonocore G, Carnielli V, De Curtis M, Darmaun D, Decsi T, et al. Enteral nutrient supply for preterm infants: commentary from the European Society of Paediatric Gastroenterology, Hepatology and Nutrition Committee on Nutrition. J Pediatr Gastroenterol Nutr. 2010;50(1):85–91. https://doi.org/10.1097/MPG.0b013e3181adaee0.
29. Goldman H. Feeding and necrotizing enterocolitis. Am J Dis Child. 1980;134(6):553–5. https://doi.org/10.1001/archpedi.1980.02130180011004.
30. Berseth CL, Bisquera JA, Paje VU. Prolonging small feeding volumes early in life decreases the incidence of necrotizing enterocolitis in very low birth weight infants. Pediatrics. 2003;111(3):529–34.
31. Morgan J, Young L, McGuire W. Slow advancement of enteral feed volumes to prevent necrotising enterocolitis in very low birth weight infants. Cochrane Database Syst Rev. 2011;3:CD001241. https://doi.org/10.1002/14651858.CD001241.pub3.
32. Oddie SJ, Young L, McGuire W. Slow advancement of enteral feed volumes to prevent necrotising enterocolitis in very low birth weight infants. Cochrane Database Syst Rev. 2017;8:CD001241. https://doi.org/10.1002/14651858.CD001241.pub7.
33. Dorling J, Abbott J, Berrington J, Bosiak B, Bowler U, Boyle E, et al. Controlled trial of two incremental milk-feeding rates in preterm infants. N Engl J Med. 2019;381(15):1434–43. https://doi.org/10.1056/NEJMoa1816654.
34. Hughes C, Dowling R. Speed of onset of adaptive mucosal hypoplasia and hypofunction in the intestine of parenterally fed rats. Clin Sci. 1980;59(5):317–27. https://doi.org/10.1042/cs0590317.
35. Darmaun D, Lapillonne A, Simeoni U, Picaud J, Rozé J, Saliba E, et al. Parenteral nutrition for preterm infants: issues and strategy. Arch Pediatr. 2018;25(4):286–94. https://doi.org/10.1016/j.arcped.2018.02.005.
36. Flidel-Rimon O, Branski D, Shinwell E. The fear of necrotizing enterocolitis versus achieving optimal growth in preterm infants—an opinion. Acta Paediatr. 2006;95(11):1341–4. https://doi.org/10.1080/08035250600719713.
37. Ozkan H, Oren H, Erdag N, Cevik N. Breast milk versus infant formulas: effects on intestinal blood flow in neonates. Indian J Pediatr. 1994;61(6):703–9. https://doi.org/10.1007/bf02751984.
38. Martinussen M, Brubakk A, Linker D, Vik T, Yao A. Mesenteric blood flow velocity and its relation to circulatory adaptation during the first week of life in healthy term infants. Pediatr Res. 1994;36(3):334–9. https://doi.org/10.1203/00006450-199409000-00011.
39. Maruyama K, Fujiu T, Inoue T, Koizumi A, Inoue F. Feeding interval and postprandial intestinal blood flow in premature infants. Pediatr Int. 2013;55(4):472–6. https://doi.org/10.1111/ped.12106.

40. Downard CD, Grant SN, Matheson PJ, Guillaume AW, Debski R, Fallat ME, Garrison RN. Altered intestinal microcirculation is the critical event in the development of necrotizing enterocolitis. J Pediatr Surg. 2011;46(6):1023–8. https://doi.org/10.1016/j.jpedsurg.2011.03.023.
41. Lee JS, Polin RA. Treatment and prevention of necrotizing enterocolitis. Semin Neonatal. 2003;8(6):449–59. https://doi.org/10.1016/s1084-2756(03)00123-4.
42. Lin J. Too much short chain fatty acids cause neonatal necrotizing enterocolitis. Med Hypotheses. 2004;62(2):291–3. https://doi.org/10.1016/s0306-9877(03)00333-5.
43. Lin J, Nafday SM, Chauvin SN, Magid MS, Pabbatireddy S, Holzman IR, Babyatsky MW. Variable effects of short chain fatty acids and lactic acid in inducing intestinal mucosal injury in newborn rats. J Pediatr Gastroenterol Nutr. 2002;35(4):545–50.
44. Pearson F, Johnson M, Leaf A. Milk osmolality: does it matter? Arch Dis Child Fetal Neonatal Ed. 2013;98(2):F166–9. https://doi.org/10.1136/adc.2011.300492.
45. Ellis Z, Tan H, Embleton N, Sangild P, van Elburg R. Milk feed osmolality and adverse events in newborn infants and animals: a systematic review. Arch Dis Child Fetal Neonatal Ed. 2019;104(3):F333–40. https://doi.org/10.1136/archdischild-2018-315946.
46. Good M, Sodhi CP, Egan CE, Afrazi A, Jia H, Yamaguchi Y, et al. Breast milk protects against the development of necrotizing enterocolitis through inhibition of Toll-like receptor 4 in the intestinal epithelium via activation of the epidermal growth factor receptor. Mucosal Immunol. 2015;8(5):1166–79. https://doi.org/10.1038/mi.2015.30.
47. Gopalakrishna KP, Macadangdang BR, Rogers MB, Tometich JT, Firek BA, Baker R, et al. Maternal IgA protects against the development of necrotizing enterocolitis in preterm infants. Nat Med. 2019;25(7):1110–5. https://doi.org/10.1038/s41591-019-0480-9.
48. Ballance WA, Dahms BB, Shenker N, Kliegman RM. Pathology of neonatal necrotizing enterocolitis: a ten-year experience. J Pediatr. 1990;117(1 Pt 2):S6–13.
49. Petrosyan M, Guner YS, Williams M, Grishin A, Ford HR. Current concepts regarding the pathogenesis of necrotizing enterocolitis. Pediatr Surg Int. 2009;25(4):309–18. https://doi.org/10.1007/s00383-009-2344-8.
50. Engel R, Virnig N, Hunt C, Levitt M. Origin of mural gas in NEC. Pediatr Res. 1973;42:292.
51. Peter CS, Feuerhahn M, Bohnhorst B, Schlaud M, Ziesing S, von der Hardt H, Poets CF. Necrotising enterocolitis: is there a relationship to specific pathogens? Eur J Pediatr. 1999;158(1):67–70.
52. Mshana SE, Gerwing L, Minde M, Hain T, Domann E, Lyamuya E, et al. Outbreak of a novel Enterobacter sp. carrying blaCTX-M-15 in a neonatal unit of a tertiary care hospital in Tanzania. Int J Antimicrob Agents. 2011;38(3):265–9. https://doi.org/10.1016/j.ijantimicag.2011.05.009.
53. Coggins SA, Wynn JL, Weitkamp JH. Infectious causes of necrotizing enterocolitis. Clin Perinatol. 2015;42(1):133–54., , ix. https://doi.org/10.1016/j.clp.2014.10.012.
54. Terrin G, Scipione A, De Curtis M. Update in pathogenesis and prospective in treatment of necrotizing enterocolitis. Biomed Res Int. 2014;2014:543765. https://doi.org/10.1155/2014/543765.
55. Remon J, Amin S, Mehendale S, Rao R, Luciano A, Garzon S, Maheshwari A. Depth of bacterial invasion in resected intestinal tissue predicts mortality in surgical necrotizing enterocolitis. J Perinatol. 2015;35(9):755–62. https://doi.org/10.1038/jp.2015.51.
56. Frost B, Caplan M. Necrotizing enterocolitis: pathophysiology, platelet-activating factor, and probiotics. Semin Pediatr Surg. 2013;22(2):88–93. https://doi.org/10.1053/j.sempedsurg.2013.01.005.
57. Cho SX, Berger PJ, Nold-Petry CA, Nold MF. The immunological landscape in necrotising enterocolitis. Expert Rev Mol Med. 2016;18:e12. https://doi.org/10.1017/erm.2016.13.
58. Leaphart CL, Cavallo J, Gribar SC, Cetin S, Li J, Branca MF, et al. A critical role for TLR4 in the pathogenesis of necrotizing enterocolitis by modulating intestinal injury and repair. J Immunol. 2007;179(7):4808–20.
59. Sodhi CP, Neal MD, Siggers R, Sho S, Ma C, Branca MF, et al. Intestinal epithelial toll-like receptor 4 regulates goblet cell development and is required for necrotizing enterocolitis in mice. Gastroenterology. 2012;143(3):708–718.e5. https://doi.org/10.1053/j.gastro.2012.05.053.

60. Mara M, Good M, Weitkamp J. Innate and adaptive immunity in necrotizing enterocolitis. Semin Fetal Neonatal Med. 2018;23(6):394–9. https://doi.org/10.1016/j.siny.2018.08.002.
61. Lu P, Sodhi C, Hackam D. Toll-like receptor regulation of intestinal development and inflammation in the pathogenesis of necrotizing enterocolitis. Pathophysiology. 2014;21(1):81–93. https://doi.org/10.1016/j.pathophys.2013.11.007.
62. Nanthakumar N, Meng D, Goldstein A, Zhu W, Lu L, Uauy R, et al. The mechanism of excessive intestinal inflammation in necrotizing enterocolitis: an immature innate immune response. PLoS One. 2011;6(3):e17776. https://doi.org/10.1371/journal.pone.0017776.
63. Neal M, Sodhi C, Dyer M, Craig B, Good M, Jia H, et al. A critical role for TLR4 induction of autophagy in the regulation of enterocyte migration and the pathogenesis of necrotizing enterocolitis. J Immunol. 2013;190(7):3541–51. https://doi.org/10.4049/jimmunol.1202264.
64. Afrazi A, Branca M, Sodhi C, Good M, Yamaguchi Y, Egan C, et al. Toll-like receptor 4-mediated endoplasmic reticulum stress in intestinal crypts induces necrotizing enterocolitis. J Biol Chem. 2014;289(14):9584–99. https://doi.org/10.1074/jbc.M113.526517.
65. Medzhitov R. Approaching the asymptote: 20 years later. Immunity. 2009;30(6):766–75. https://doi.org/10.1016/j.immuni.2009.06.004.
66. Yang J, Zhao Y, Shao F. Non-canonical activation of inflammatory caspases by cytosolic LPS in innate immunity. Curr Opin Immunol. 2015;32:78–83. https://doi.org/10.1016/j.coi.2015.01.007.
67. Guijarro-Muñoz I, Compte M, Álvarez-Cienfuegos A, Álvarez-Vallina L, Sanz L. Lipopolysaccharide activates toll-like receptor 4 (TLR4)-mediated NF-κB signaling pathway and proinflammatory response in human pericytes. J Biol Chem. 2014;289(4):2457–68. https://doi.org/10.1074/jbc.M113.521161.
68. Caplan M, Sun X, Hseuh W, Hageman J. Role of platelet activating factor and tumor necrosis factor-alpha in neonatal necrotizing enterocolitis. J Pediatr. 1990;116(6):960–4. https://doi.org/10.1016/s0022-3476(05)80661-4.
69. Gonzalez-Crussi F, Hsueh W. Experimental model of ischemic bowel necrosis. the role of platelet-activating factor and endotoxin. Am J Pathol. 1983;112(1):127–35.
70. Furukawa M, Lee E, Johnston J. Platelet-activating factor-induced ischemic bowel necrosis: the effect of platelet-activating factor acetylhydrolase. Pediatr Res. 1993;34(2):237–41. https://doi.org/10.1203/00006450-199308000-00027.
71. Caplan M, Hedlund E, Adler L, Lickerman M, Hsueh W. The platelet-activating factor receptor antagonist WEB 2170 prevents neonatal necrotizing enterocolitis in rats. J Pediatr Gastroenterol Nutr. 1997;24(3):296–301. https://doi.org/10.1097/00005176-199703000-00012.
72. Caplan M, Lickerman M, Adler L, Dietsch G, Yu A. The role of recombinant platelet-activating factor acetylhydrolase in a neonatal rat model of necrotizing enterocolitis. Pediatr Res. 1997;42(6):779–83. https://doi.org/10.1203/00006450-199712000-00010.
73. Moya F, Eguchi H, Zhao B, Furukawa M, Sfeir J, Osorio M, et al. Platelet-activating factor acetylhydrolase in term and preterm human milk: a preliminary report. J Pediatr Gastroenterol Nutr. 1994;19(2):236–9. https://doi.org/10.1097/00005176-199408000-00015.
74. Soliman A, Michelsen K, Karahashi H, Lu J, Meng F, Qu X, et al. Platelet-activating factor induces TLR4 expression in intestinal epithelial cells: implication for the pathogenesis of necrotizing enterocolitis. PLoS One. 2010;5(10):e15044. https://doi.org/10.1371/journal.pone.0015044.
75. Musemeche C, Caplan M, Hsueh W, Sun X, Kelly A. Experimental necrotizing enterocolitis: the role of polymorphonuclear neutrophils. J Pediatr Surg. 1991;26(9):1047–9. https://doi.org/10.1016/0022-3468(91)90671-f.
76. Emami C, Mittal R, Wang L, Ford H, Prasadarao N. Role of neutrophils and macrophages in the pathogenesis of necrotizing enterocolitis caused by cronobacter sakazakii. J Surg Res. 2012;172(1):18–28. https://doi.org/10.1016/j.jss.2011.04.019.
77. Christensen R, Yoder B, Baer V, Snow G, Butler A. Early-onset neutropenia in small-for-gestational-age infants. Pediatrics. 2015;136(5):e1259–67. https://doi.org/10.1542/peds.2015-1638.

78. Aquino E, Neves A, Santos K, Uribe C, Souza P, Correa J, et al. Proteomic analysis of neutrophil priming by PAF. Protein Pept Lett. 2016;23(2):142–51. https://doi.org/10.217 4/0929866523666151202210604.
79. Bain C, Schridde A. Origin, differentiation, and function of intestinal macrophages. Front Immunol. 2018;9:2733. https://doi.org/10.3389/fimmu.2018.02733.
80. Bain C, Scott C, Uronen-Hansson H, Gudjonsson S, Jansson O, Grip O, et al. Resident and pro-inflammatory macrophages in the colon represent alternative context-dependent fates of the same Ly6Chi monocyte precursors. Mucosal Immunol. 2013;6(3):498–510. https://doi.org/10.1038/mi.2012.89.
81. Smythies L, Sellers M, Clements R, Mosteller-Barnum M, Meng G, Benjamin W, et al. Human Intestinal macrophages display profound inflammatory anergy despite avid phagocytic and bacteriocidal activity. J Clin Invest. 2005;115(1):66–75. https://doi.org/10.1172/JCI19229.
82. MohanKumar K, Namachivayam K, Chapalamadugu K, Garzon S, Premkumar M, Tipparaju S, Maheshwari A. Smad7 interrupts TGF-β signaling in intestinal macrophages and promotes inflammatory activation of these cells during necrotizing enterocolitis. Pediatr Res. 2016;79(6):951–61. https://doi.org/10.1038/pr.2016.18.
83. MohanKumar K, Kaza N, Jagadeeswaran R, Garzon S, Bansal A, Kurundkar A, et al. Gut mucosal injury in neonates is marked by macrophage infiltration in contrast to pleomorphic infiltrates in adult: evidence from an animal model. Am J Physiol Gastrointest Liver Physiol. 2012;303(1):G93–102. https://doi.org/10.1152/ajpgi.00016.2012.
84. Maheshwari A, Kelly DR, Nicola T, Ambalavanan N, Jain SK, Murphy-Ullrich J, et al. TGF-beta2 suppresses macrophage cytokine production and mucosal inflammatory responses in the developing intestine. Gastroenterology. 2011;140(1):242–53. https://doi.org/10.1053/j.gastro.2010.09.043.
85. Gibbons D, Haque S, Silberzahn T, Hamilton K, Langford C, Ellis P, et al. Neonates harbour highly active gammadelta T cells with selective impairments in preterm infants. Eur J Immunol. 2009;39(7):1794–806. https://doi.org/10.1002/eji.200939222.
86. Weitkamp J, Rosen M, Zhao Z, Koyama T, Geem D, Denning T, et al. Small intestinal intraepithelial TCRγδ+ T lymphocytes are present in the premature intestine but selectively reduced in surgical necrotizing enterocolitis. PLoS One. 2014;9(6):e99042. https://doi.org/10.1371/journal.pone.0099042.
87. Egan C, Sodhi C, Good M, Lin J, Jia H, Yamaguchi Y, et al. Toll-like receptor 4-mediated lymphocyte influx induces neonatal necrotizing enterocolitis. J Clin Investig. 2016;126(2):495–508. https://doi.org/10.1172/JCI83356.
88. Zani A, Pierro A. Necrotizing enterocolitis: controversies and challenges. F1000Res. 2015;4:F1000. https://doi.org/10.12688/f1000research.6888.1.
89. Llanos A, Moss M, Pinzòn M, Dye T, Sinkin R, Kendig J. Epidemiology of neonatal necrotising enterocolitis: a population-based study. Paediatr Perinat Epidemiol. 2002;16(4):342–9. https://doi.org/10.1046/j.1365-3016.2002.00445.x.
90. Uauy R, Fanaroff A, Korones S, Phillips E, Phillips J, Wright L. Necrotizing enterocolitis in very low birth weight infants: biodemographic and clinical correlates. National Institute of Child Health and Human Development Neonatal Research Network. J Pediatr. 1991;119(4):630–8. https://doi.org/10.1016/s0022-3476(05)82418-7.
91. Bhandari V, Bizzarro M, Shetty A, Zhong X, Page G, Zhang H, et al. Familial and genetic susceptibility to major neonatal morbidities in preterm twins. Pediatrics. 2006;117(6):1901–6. https://doi.org/10.1542/peds.2005-1414.
92. Cuna A, George L, Sampath V. Genetic predisposition to necrotizing enterocolitis in premature infants: current knowledge, challenges, and future directions. Semin Fetal Neonatal Med. 2018;23(6):387–93. https://doi.org/10.1016/j.siny.2018.08.006.
93. Kalogeris T, Baines CP, Krenz M, Korthuis RJ. Cell biology of ischemia/reperfusion injury. Int Rev Cell Mol Biol. 2012;298:229–317. https://doi.org/10.1016/b978-0-12-394309-5.00006-7.
94. Jennings RB, Sommers HM, Smyth GA, Flack HA, Linn H. Myocardial necrosis induced by temporary occlusion of a coronary artery in the dog. Arch Pathol. 1960;70:68–78.

95. Askie L, Darlow B, Davis P, Finer N, Stenson B, Vento M, Whyte R. Effects of targeting lower versus higher arterial oxygen saturations on death or disability in preterm infants. Cochrane Database Syst Rev. 2017;4(4):CD011190. https://doi.org/10.1002/14651858. CD011190.pub2.

96. Lloyd JR. The etiology of gastrointestinal perforations in the newborn. J Pediatr Surg. 1969;4(1):77–84.

97. Caplan M, Fanaroff A. Necrotizing: a historical perspective. Semin Perinatol. 2017;41(1):2–6. https://doi.org/10.1053/j.semperi.2016.09.012.

98. Nankervis CA, Giannone PJ, Reber KM. The neonatal intestinal vasculature: contributing factors to necrotizing enterocolitis. Semin Perinatol. 2008;32(2):83–91. https://doi.org/10.1053/j.semperi.2008.01.003.

99. Chen Y, Chang KT, Lian DW, Lu H, Roy S, Laksmi NK, et al. The role of ischemia in necrotizing enterocolitis. J Pediatr Surg. 2016;51(8):1255–61. https://doi.org/10.1016/j.jpedsurg.2015.12.015.

100. Huang LE, Arany Z, Livingston DM, Bunn HF. Activation of hypoxia-inducible transcription factor depends primarily upon redox-sensitive stabilization of its alpha subunit. J Biol Chem. 1996;271(50):32253–9. https://doi.org/10.1074/jbc.271.50.32253.

101. Fang S, Kempley ST, Gamsu HR. Prediction of early tolerance to enteral feeding in preterm infants by measurement of superior mesenteric artery blood flow velocity. Arch Dis Child Fetal Neonatal Ed. 2001;85(1):F42–5.

102. Murdoch EM, Sinha AK, Shanmugalingam ST, Smith GC, Kempley ST. Doppler flow velocimetry in the superior mesenteric artery on the first day of life in preterm infants and the risk of neonatal necrotizing enterocolitis. Pediatrics. 2006;118(5):1999–2003. https://doi.org/10.1542/peds.2006-0272.

103. Polin RA, Pollack PF, Barlow B, Wigger HJ, Slovis TL, Santulli TV, Heird WC. Necrotizing enterocolitis in term infants. J Pediatr. 1976;89(3):460–2.

104. Chen Y, Koike Y, Miyake H, Li B, Lee C, Hock A, et al. Formula feeding and systemic hypoxia synergistically induce intestinal hypoxia in experimental necrotizing enterocolitis. Pediatr Surg Int. 2016;32(12):1115–9. https://doi.org/10.1007/s00383-016-3997-8.

105. Yazji I, Sodhi CP, Lee EK, Good M, Egan CE, Afrazi A, et al. Endothelial TLR4 activation impairs intestinal microcirculatory perfusion in necrotizing enterocolitis via eNOS-NO-nitrite signaling. Proc Natl Acad Sci U S A. 2013;110(23):9451–6. https://doi.org/10.1073/pnas.1219997110.

106. Neu J, Modi N, Caplan M. Necrotizing enterocolitis comes in different forms: historical perspectives and defining the disease. Semin Fetal Neonatal Med. 2018;23(6):370–3. https://doi.org/10.1016/j.siny.2018.07.004.

107. Maayan-Metzger A, Itzchak A, Mazkereth R, Kuint J. Necrotizing enterocolitis in full-term infants: case-control study and review of the literature. J Perinatol. 2004;24(8):494–9. https://doi.org/10.1038/sj.jp.7211135.

108. McElhinney DB, Hedrick HL, Bush DM, Pereira GR, Stafford PW, Gaynor JW, et al. Necrotizing enterocolitis in neonates with congenital heart disease: risk factors and outcomes. Pediatrics. 2000;106(5):1080–7.

109. Bernstein I, Horbar J, Badger G, Ohlsson A, Golan A. Morbidity and mortality among very-low-birth-weight neonates with intrauterine growth restriction. The Vermont Oxford Network. Am J Obstet Gynecol. 2000;182(1 Pt 1):198–206. https://doi.org/10.1016/s0002-9378(00)70513-8.

110. Kiserud T, Ebbing C, Kessler J, Rasmussen S. Fetal cardiac output, distribution to the placenta and impact of placental compromise. Ultrasound Obstet Gynecol. 2006;28(2):126–36. https://doi.org/10.1002/uog.2832.

111. Alfirevic Z, Neilson J. WITHDRAWN. Doppler ultrasound for fetal assessment in high risk pregnancies. Cochrane Database Syst Rev. 2010;2010(1):CD000073. https://doi.org/10.1002/14651858.CD000073.pub2.

112. Westby Eger S, Kessler J, Kiserud T, Markestad T, Sommerfelt K. Foetal Doppler abnormality is associated with increased risk of sepsis and necrotising enterocolitis in preterm infants. Acta Paediatr. 2015;104(4):368–76. https://doi.org/10.1111/apa.12893.

113. Tewari V, Dubey S, Kumar R, Vardhan S, Sreedhar C, Gupta G. Early versus late enteral feeding in preterm intrauterine growth restricted neonates with antenatal Doppler abnormalities: an open-label randomized trial. J Trop Pediatr. 2018;64(1):4–14. https://doi.org/10.1093/tropej/fmx018.
114. Hay S, Zupancic J, Flannery D, Kirpalani H, Dukhovny D. Should we believe in transfusion-associated enterocolitis? Applying a GRADE to the literature. Semin Perinatol. 2017;41(1):80–91. https://doi.org/10.1053/j.semperi.2016.09.021.
115. Blau J, Calo JM, Dozor D, Sutton M, Alpan G, La Gamma EF. Transfusion-related acute gut injury: necrotizing enterocolitis in very low birth weight neonates after packed red blood cell transfusion. J Pediatr. 2011;158(3):403–9. https://doi.org/10.1016/j.jpeds.2010.09.015.
116. Janjindamai W, Prapruettrong A, Thatrimontrichai A, Dissaneevate S, Maneenil G, Geater A. Risk of necrotizing enterocolitis following packed red blood cell transfusion in very low birth weight infants. Indian J Pediatr. 2019;86(4):347–53. https://doi.org/10.1007/s12098-019-02887-7.
117. Patel RM, Knezevic A, Shenvi N, Hinkes M, Keene S, Roback JD, et al. Association of red blood cell transfusion, anemia, and necrotizing enterocolitis in very low-birth-weight infants. JAMA. 2016;315(9):889–97. https://doi.org/10.1001/jama.2016.1204.
118. Maheshwari A, Patel R, Christensen R. Anemia, red blood cell transfusions, and necrotizing enterocolitis. Semin Pediatr Surg. 2018;27(1):47–51. https://doi.org/10.1053/j.sempedsurg.2017.11.009.
119. Szabo J, Mayfield S, Oh W, Stonestreet B. Postprandial gastrointestinal blood flow and oxygen consumption: effects of hypoxemia in neonatal piglets. Pediatr Res. 1987;21(1):93–8. https://doi.org/10.1203/00006450-198701000-00020.
120. Lee JA. Practice for preterm patent ductus arteriosus; focusing on the hemodynamic significance and the impact on the neonatal outcomes. Korean J Pediatr. 2019;62(7):245–51. https://doi.org/10.3345/kjp.2018.07213.
121. Rolland A, Shankar-Aguilera S, Diomande D, Zupan-Simunek V, Boileau P. Natural evolution of patent ductus arteriosus in the extremely preterm infant. Arch Dis Child Fetal Neonatal Ed. 2015;100(1):F55–8. https://doi.org/10.1136/archdischild-2014-306339.
122. Heuchan AM, Clyman RI. Managing the patent ductus arteriosus: current treatment options. Arch Dis Child Fetal Neonatal Ed. 2014;99(5):F431–6. https://doi.org/10.1136/archdischild-2014-306176.
123. Ledo A, Aguar M, Nunez-Ramiro A, Saenz P, Vento M. Abdominal near-infrared spectroscopy detects low mesenteric perfusion early in preterm infants with hemodynamic significant ductus arteriosus. Neonatology. 2017;112(3):238–45. https://doi.org/10.1159/000475933.
124. Kort E. Patent ductus arteriosus in the preterm infant: an update on morbidity and mortality. Curr Pediatr Rev. 2016;12(2):98–105. https://doi.org/10.2174/1573396312021605060011621.
125. Ezenwa B, Pena E, Schlegel A, Bapat R, Shepherd EG, Nelin LD. Effects of practice change on outcomes of extremely preterm infants with patent ductus arteriosus. Acta Paediatr. 2019;108(1):88–93. https://doi.org/10.1111/apa.14423.
126. Mitra S, Florez I, Tamayo M, Mbuagbaw L, Vanniyasingam T, Veroniki A, et al. Association of placebo, indomethacin, ibuprofen, and acetaminophen with closure of hemodynamically significant patent ductus arteriosus in preterm infants: a systematic review and meta-analysis. JAMA. 2018;319(12):1221–38. https://doi.org/10.1001/jama.2018.1896.
127. Yellon DM, Hausenloy DJ. Myocardial reperfusion injury. N Engl J Med. 2007;357(11):1121–35. https://doi.org/10.1056/NEJMra071667.
128. Young CM, Kingma SD, Neu J. Ischemia-reperfusion and neonatal intestinal injury. J Pediatr. 2011;158(2 Suppl):e25–8. https://doi.org/10.1016/j.jpeds.2010.11.009.
129. Sanada S, Komuro I, Kitakaze M. Pathophysiology of myocardial reperfusion injury: preconditioning, postconditioning, and translational aspects of protective measures. Am J Physiol Heart Circ Physiol. 2011;301(5):H1723–41. https://doi.org/10.1152/ajpheart.00553.2011.
130. Bowker R, Yan X, De Plaen I. Intestinal microcirculation and necrotizing enterocolitis: the vascular endothelial growth factor system. Semin Fetal Neonatal Med. 2018;23(6):411–5. https://doi.org/10.1016/j.siny.2018.08.008.

Chapter 6
Preventing Necrotising Enterocolitis

Contents

Abstract Necrotising enterocolitis is a devastating disease. The treatments for NEC are limited and outcomes remain poor. As such, the imperative to prevent NEC is very strong. Unfortunately there are few effective options. There is undoubtedly a need for novel interventions that reduce the risk of infants developing NEC.

NEC is primarily a disease of premature infants. As such, the most effective way to prevent NEC is to prevent premature birth. This has been a long term aim for obstetric care but despite extensive research and multiple potential interventions, the rates of premature birth are static or possibly rising.

© The Author(s), under exclusive license to Springer Nature
Switzerland AG 2024
I. Jones, *Necrotising Enterocolitis in Clinical Practice*, In Clinical Practice,
https://doi.org/10.1007/978-3-031-64148-0_6

The routine use of antenatal steroids for lung maturation has the addition benefit of reducing the risk of NEC. Probiotics administration to infants remains controversial. There is some evidence of effectiveness but multiple studies have produced conflicting results. The most recent evidence suggests that the rate of feed advancement probably is not a factor in NEC but the choice of milk undoubtedly is. Maternal milk is the safest option with the lowest risk of NEC but donor milk is significantly better that cows' milk-based formula feeds and arguably is not used enough in routine practice.

Keywords NEC prevention strategies · Breastfeeding and NEC prevention Human milk fortification · Donor human milk in NEC prevention · Exclusive human milk diet · Probiotics for NEC prevention · Prebiotics for NEC prevention Synbiotics for NEC prevention · Antibiotic stewardship in NEC prevention · Early feeding initiation · Slow advancement of enteral feeds · Trophic feeds in NEC prevention · Minimizing exposure to harmful bacteria · Avoidance of unnecessary antibiotics · Aseptic techniques in neonatal care · Multidisciplinary NEC prevention protocols · NEC screening protocols · Reduced use of acid-suppressive medications · Minimally invasive surgical techniques in preterm infants Enhanced parenteral nutrition strategies

6.1 Introduction

The very commonly used cliché states that *prevention is better than cure*. This truism applies to so many circumstances. It is especially true when the treatment options are very limited: when the putative 'cure' either does not exist or is often not effective. It is especially true when the outcomes are poor.

The following two chapters focus on current management of NEC. Chapter 9 describes outcomes. The summary of these is depressingly simple: treatment of NEC is essentially supportive only unless the babies need surgery. Outcomes are poor, especially for those that need surgery.

Therefore there is a significant imperative to prevent NEC. Novel treatments have not been forthcoming in several decades and outcomes are potentially no better than they were in the 1980s.

The search for preventative strategies in NEC has not been as fruitless as the hunt for new treatments but the effective options remain limited.

6.2 Prematurity

It is a fairly banal statement but given that NEC is a disease of prematurity, the most effective way to prevent NEC is to prevent pre-term birth. This is so easy to say but current data suggests that preterm birth rates have risen in the first decade of the twenty-first century, rather than falling and then become static since 2010. This is despite good evidence of cost-effective interventions that do reduce the risk of premature labour.

The World Health Organisation estimates that there were 13.4 million babies born prematurely in 2020 [1] and complications due to prematurity is the leading cause of death among children under 5 years of age [2]. Most tellingly, it is likely that three-quarters of these 900,000 deaths could be prevented with current cost-effective interventions.

6.2.1 Rates of Prematurity Across the World

The number of pre-term births (defined as birth prior to 37 weeks completed gestation) varies quite dramatically between countries, with more than half occurring in just eight countries; namely India, Pakistan, Nigeria, China, Ethiopia, Bangladesh, Democratic Republic of Congo, and USA. The high total numbers partly reflect large populations, which is why China appears in this list with 750,000 premature births. This is similar to the total number of live births in the UK. It reflects though, a rate of pre-term birth of only 6.1% which is much lower than the international average and less than half the rate recorded in Pakistan of 14%.

Table 6.1 shows the premature birth rate by region with figures from 2010 and 2020 which demonstrates how overall the rates are essentially static. It should be noted that there are significant variations between countries across the world with some seeing rising rates and others failing.

More importantly for our purposes here with NEC, there has not been a significant fall in preterm birth rates. Despite decades of research, the hope of achieving a meaningful reduction in pre-term birth—and therefore a reduction in the complications of pre-term birth—seems as far off as it did in the mid-1980s [3]. In the following section, effective ways of preventing preterm birth will be discussed. There is good evidence that these measures can work but for whatever reason, this has not translated so far into a real world difference. It does remain however, arguably the best strategy for preventing NEC.

Table 6.1 Global estimates of preterm birth rates

Region	Estimated rate of premature birth %	
	2010	2020
Southern Asia	13.3	13.2
Sub-Saharan Africa	10.1	10.1
Western Asia, Northern Africa	8.8	9.1
North America, Australia, New Zealand, Central Asia and Europe	7.8	7.9
Eastern Asia, South-eastern Asia and Oceania	6.6	6.8
Worldwide	**9.8**	**9.9**

Based on Ohuma et al. (2023) [1]

6.2.2 Strategies to Reduce Pre-term Delivery

"Pre-term birth" is not really a diagnosis as it is a catch-all term for any baby born before 37 weeks completed gestation. Prematurity is a result of multiple different pathways. Some of the causes are amenable to intervention whilst others are much less so. There is evidence (of various levels) for each of the following [4] as effective ways to reduce the number of pre-term births:

- Prevent non-medically indicated late preterm birth
- Progesterone supplementation
- Cervical cerclage
- Reduce tobacco consumption in pregnancy
- Judicious use of fertility treatments
- Dedicated preterm birth prevention clinics

These methods of preventing preterm labour are briefly discussed in turn, below.

6.2.2.1 Preventing Non-medically Indicated Later Preterm Birth

Late pre-term birth refers to babies born between 34 and 36 weeks, 6 days gestation. Between 1990 and 2006, the rate of delivery in this group went up by 20% in the USA and by similar amounts in other developed countries.

These births are often medically induced or birth by c-section due to concerns about maternal or foetal well-being. This therefore represents a very heterogenous group. There are inevitable confounders when looking at outcomes—i.e. these babies (or their mothers) have medical concerns when birth occurs. This means that it is difficult to derive good evidence on this kind of decision-making. The rise in the rate of babies being born at this gestation without a conconment fall in still-birth suggests that overall there is a need for a change in strategies and protocols. The beneficial effect is not really being achieved as a cost of an increased risk of complications due to prematurity. This can be very difficult as each individual case can only ever be judged on its own merits.

From a global health perspective there is a lot of potential to reduce pre-term birth here, despite the difficulties. However from an NEC point of view, this is probably of only minor importance as these late pre-term group are at relatively low risk of NEC.

6.2.2.2 Progesterone Supplementation

There is good evidence that progesterone supplementation during pregnancy can prevent pre-term birth although the exact mechanisms by which is works remains unknown. Progesterone can be given orally, intravenously or vaginally.

In women with a past history of pre-term birth, progesterone treatment reduces the risk of birth before 34 weeks by two thirds and the risk of birth before 37 weeks by nearly half. Similarly the risk of perinatal death is halved [5]. There is also evidence of a benefit in women found to have a short cervix in mid pregnancy and several studies suggest that progesterone can be effective at delaying delivery in women who have had an episode of threatened pre-term labour.

6.2.2.3 Cervical Cerclage

Cervical cerclage was first described in the 1950s and means the surgical placement of a suture or tape around the cervix in an attempt to prevent dilatation and consequential preterm birth. It is often used for so-called incompetence cervix, especially when associated with previous preterm labour. Meta-analysis of randomised control trials has shown that this results in a 20% reduction in pre-term labour [4].

6.2.2.4 Reduce Tobacco Consumption in Pregnancy

Tobacco smoking in pregnancy causes preterm birth and there is a dose-related relationship between consumption and reduction in birthweight. Second-hand smoke has also been shown to have an association with an increased risk of still birth, preterm birth and low birthweight.

In high-income countries, rates of smoking in pregnancy have declined overall but this decline has not been seen in all socioeconomic groups [4].

6.2.2.5 Judicious Use of Fertility Treatments

In-vitro fertilisation (IVF) is strongly associated with multiple births. Indeed from 1972 to 2011, the rate of multiple birth in the USA nearly doubled from 1.8% to 3.5%. This rise was entirely attributed to medically assisted reproduction as the rate of natural multiple conception remained unchanged. Gestation is shorter in multiple pregnancies and birthweights are lower. As well as IVF, less invasive treatments such as ovarian stimulation can also result in multiple pregnancy.

In the early days of IVF, it was common practice to implant multiple embryos to maximise the chance of successful pregnancy. More recently, single embryo transfer has become widely accepted in many countries.

The majority of European countries now report a single embryo transfer rate of more than 50% [6]. The rate of multiple births with IVF in the UK has now fallen to 5% in 2021 from a peak of nearly 30% in the early 1990s [7].

6.2.2.6 Dedicated Preterm Birth Prevention Clinics

There is some evidence that dedicated clinics that enable a multidisciplinary and multifaceted approach can be effective at reducing pre-term births. It is not surprising that the multitude of causes of prematurity require a diverse range of interventions and that a dedicated clinic can be the best way to coordinate a diverse response. Data from such clinics in the USA has shown a potential to reduce preterm birth by a quarter although, as yet there is limited evidence of this success being widely reproduced.

6.2.2.7 Other Interventions That May Reduce the Risk of Preterm Birth

It has long been recognised that preterm labour is associated with leucocytosis of the amniotic fluid secondary to invasion of various bacteria such as *Ureaplasma urealyticum, Mycoplasma hominis, Gardnerella vaginalis*, peptostreptococci, and bacteroides species. Currently there is a no clear evidence of how to identify and treat such infections and no data on how that by doing so, preterm labour can be reduced [8]. It is certainly logical to assume that identifying and treating such infections could be effective but currently there is no evidence of how to do this nor that doing so would be as effective as hoped.

Maternal nutrition is a recognised risk factor as a low maternal body mass index (BMI) pre-pregnancy is associated with an increased risk of preterm birth and obesity appears to be protective. Translating that into a strategy to improve maternal health and prevent preterm labour has yet to bear fruit.

There are several studies that report high levels of maternal psychological or social stress are associated with preterm labour, however so far trials of interventions to alleviate maternal stress have not resulted in reduced rates of preterm delivery.

Cervical cancer can be a very aggressive disease and often fatal in young women. Cervical screening programs that identified and treated cervical intra-epithelial neoplasia (CIN) have saved many lives. However, women who have had treatment for CIN are at a higher risk of preterm delivery. The widespread introduction of HPV vaccinations will no doubt lead to a significant reduction in women needing treatment for CIN and a reduction in mortality. An additional benefit is that because fewer women will need invasive treatment of CIN there will be likely be a reduced risk of preterm birth for these women.

6.3 Antenatal Corticosteroids

Antenatal steroids for threatened preterm labour is now standard practice in many countries. It was first discovered by Liggins in sheep experiments in 1969 that the administration of corticosteroids to ewes just prior to delivery had a dramatic effect on the maturation of the lamb's lungs. Liggins described inflation in the lungs of lambs born at gestations when the lungs would be expected to be airless [9, 10]. The first human randomised control trial followed in 1972 [9].

Respiratory distress syndrome (RDS) is a serious complication of preterm birth. As discussed in Chap. 2, the routine administration of surfactant resulted in a large step-change in the outcomes of premature babies. It addition, corticosteroids given to mothers prior to delivery has been shown to further decrease the risk of RDS and improve outcomes.

The updated Cochrane review shows that administration of a single course of corticosteroids reduced perinatal death by around a quarter, neonatal death by a third, and moderate to severe RDS by nearly half [10].

The same review also concluded, based on ten studies with nearly 5000 infants, that administration of antenatal steroids halved the risk of NEC (Risk ratio: 0.50 (95% C.I.: 0.32–0.78)). The primary indication for the use of steroids is for lung maturation and the benefit in respiratory function but there is clearly also a marked benefit in terms of preventing NEC as well.

The Royal College of Obstetrics and Gynaecology guidelines recommends [11]:

Corticosteroids should be offered to women between 24 + 0 and 34 + 6 weeks' gestation in whom imminent preterm birth is anticipated (either due to established preterm labour, preterm prelabour rupture of membranes [PPROM] or planned preterm birth).

The suggested protocol for administration is:

In the UK it is recommended that 24 mg dexamethasone phosphate is given intramuscularly in two divided doses of 12 mg 24 hours apart or four divided doses of 6 mg 12 hours apart

As steroid administration was introduced for a completely different reason and the reduction in NEC rates was discovered as an incidental benefit, it follows that the evidence for the effectiveness predates understanding of the mechanism by which that protective effect is achieved.

A higher risk of NEC is associated with the need for intubation and ventilation. It is therefore plausible that improving lung health could result in a reduced risk of NEC as a secondary effect. That may well be part of the pathway by which antenatal steroid are protective against NEC. However there is also evidence of a more direct action.

Antenatal corticosteroids stimulate the production of surfactant-associated proteins in the lung. Surfactant proteins are not only found in the lung but also in the intestine. Work done using an animal model of NEC showed that administration of corticosteroids to mothers prior to delivery stimulated intestinal surfactant protein D (SP-D), decreased inflammatory responses and maintained intestinal barrier integrity in the new born pups [12]. There is therefore good data on the mechanisms by which corticosteroids act on the intestine and epidemiological evidence of a meaningful reduction in the risk of NEC.

In clinical practice, there are babies who are born prematurely without the administration of antenatal steroids, even in high income settings. This is usually due to a lack of antenatal care due to poor engagement with healthcare services or because of a precipitous preterm labour not allowing time for administration. In a context where steroids are routine, there is a clear implication that such infants will be at higher-risk than many of their compatriots.

6.4 Feeding Strategies

Enteral feeding is one of the most important risk factors for NEC. Furthermore there is good evidence that the choice of feed makes a big difference to the risk of NEC whilst the rate of advancement of feed does not have an effect on this risk.

6.4.1 Choice of Feed

Babies who have never been fed (for whatever reason) very rarely get NEC [13]. Babies fed on cows' milk-based formula have much higher rates of NEC than those fed on breast milk. The use of exclusive maternal breast milk reduces the risk of NEC sixfold [14]. Donor breast milk also reduces the risk but the reduction is smaller at just under threefold [15, 16].There is also a demonstrable dose effect with milk feeds whereby the risk of NEC is reduced with every 10% increase in the proportion of feed that is human milk [17]. The mechanisms by which feeding and especially formula feeding lead to NEC are discussed in detail in Chap. 5 but the epidemiological data is clear; the higher the proportion of human milk in an infant's feeding regimen, the lower the risk of NEC. Hence, arguably the most important preventative strategy in current neonatal care to reduce the risk of NEC, is the preferential use of human milk over formula.

Milk fortifiers are controversial. There is contradictory evidence as to whether fortifiers increase the risk of NEC or not. The problem is that preterm neonates cannot get sufficient nutrients from breast milk alone to grow. Milk fortifiers are based on cows' milk and thus in some ways are akin to formula feeds. Ultimately the risk of NEC must be weighed against the risks to development of inadequate growth. ESPGHAN guidelines for all infants weighing less than 1800 g advise mother's own milk as primary feed with the addition of individualised fortification as needed [18].

Human-milk-derived fortifiers are now commercially available. In the long term these may be the answer—providing sufficient nutrition to allow growth whilst minimising the exposure to cows' milk-based products. However, they are very expensive and the evidence of a clear benefit over conventional fortifiers does not currently exist.

6.4.2 Feeding Rates

The temporal relationship between the development of NEC and feeding has been clearly demonstrated. Similarly, the evidence that enteral feeding is an undoubted trigger for NEC is clear cut. Additionally the collective evidence from various animal studies shows that enteral feeding increases the metabolic demand on the intestine and this is a key pathway for the pathogenesis of NEC (Chap. 5). Taking these things together, it is logical to consider that the volume of feed given may also be important and therefore the question for clinical practice is how fast should feeds be advanced in preterm babies?

Advancing feeds more slowly results in poorer growth (with potential impact on neurodevelopment in the long term) therefore the risk of NEC from rapid feed advancement (if there indeed is one) must be balanced against the negative effect of slower feeds [19, 20].

To a large extent this question has been answered by the SIFT trial.

6.4.3 Speed of Increasing Milk Feeds Trial (SIFT) [21]

The SIFT trial recruited more than 2800 infants who were born before 32 weeks completed gestation or weighing less than 1500 g. Infants were randomised to a slower increment group or a faster increment group.

New born premature infants are routinely started on parenteral nutrition and then given milk feeds as the intestine will tolerate. 'Full enteral feeds' is typically considered to be 150 mL/kg/day. Some neonates will require larger volumes in order to grow and as described above, many will need fortifiers. In essence, the sooner enteral feeds are achieved, the better as this reduces central catheter days and sepsis risk as well as reducing the other risks of parenteral nutrition. In this trial, slower feed advancement was 18 mL/kg/day and the faster group was 30 mL/kg/day. In an infant weighing 600 g, 18 mL/kg/day equates to around 0.5 mL/h of milk feed.

SIFT showed no difference in their primary outcome of survival without severe neurodisability (at 24 months corrected age) between the two groups. The rate of NEC in both groups was around 5–6%, with no statistical difference.

Sub-group analysis did show an advantage for slower feed advancement (in terms of survival without severe disability) in neonates fed on formula alone. This is based on small numbers but would suggest more caution with formula feeds may be appropriate.

6.5 Probiotics

Probiotics are dietary supplements that contain potentially beneficial microorganisms. It has been shown that infants that develop NEC are colonised with potentially pathogenic bacteria in the days preceding the development of the disease. The evolution of the microbiome in preterm infants is not the same as in term babies and it has long been thought that the addition of probiotics could aid the development of the intestinal flora and thereby reduce the exposure to pathogenic organisms. Such a reduction could then reduce the risk of NEC. *Bifidobacterium* and *Lactobacillus* species can be given as can mixtures of *Bifidobacterium*, and *Streptococcus* species.

Detailed studies suggest that providing commensal bacteria to the preterm gut has multiple positive effects, including; strengthening of the intestinal barrier, improved peristalsis and by stimulating mucin production.

Bifidobacterium are non-motile, gram-positive anaerobes. Similarly, Lactobacillus are gram-positive, (aerotolerant) anaerobic non-spore-forming bacteria. Both of them are normal commensals of the alimentary tract of human infants, children and adults.

6.5.1 Cochrane Review and Current Guidelines

The most recent Cochrane review found that whilst the data does show a reduced risk of NEC with probiotic use, the evidence was of low to moderate quality and hence no firm recommendation can be made [22].

Allowing for those limitations, the headline figures are quite impressive. Based on nearly 60 trials in over 11,000 infants born before 32 weeks or below 1500 g, the rate of NEC in the placebo group was 6%, falling to 3.3% in the probiotic group.

The trials that have been conducted are relatively heterogeneous in terms of the specific organism or organisms used as probiotics. This is a limitation in making the findings applicable to routine practice.

Some centres have adopted protocols for routine probiotic use but not all. There have been very rare cases of sepsis associated with probiotic administration. For most infants, the literature would suggest that the risks are very low and outweighed by the potential benefit. One specific problem with probiotics is that they are a food product rather than a medicine. As such, they are subject to a very different (and less strict) regulatory framework. In essence, the issue is that probiotics contents do not always match their label precisely. One study found that only 1 out of 16 tested commercial probiotic products matched exactly the label, including probiotics marketed specifically for infants [23].

6.5.2 The Specific Challenge of Conducting Probiotic Studies

Unsurprisingly, one of the conclusions from the Cochrane review is that more, high quality trials are needed to answer this question. However, there is a specific issue with conducting trials of probiotics that makes this particularly challenging. One of the larger, well-designed blinded control studies of probiotics was published in 2016 [24]. This study involved around 1200 participants in multiple centres and used a probiotic product containing *Bifidobacterium breve*. The probiotic (or placebo) was given once a day to infants between 23 weeks 0 days completed gestation and 30 weeks and 6 days gestation. The study showed no difference in the risk of NEC between the groups. So on that basis, one might conclude that there is no benefit from giving probiotics but it is more complicated than that. This study including lots of other data and outcome measures as well. Stool samples were taken from all of the participants to test for successful colonisation with the organism, *B. breve*. The stool samples were analysed by both culture and PCR. Two weeks after birth, around 84% of the infants given probiotics had positive stool results (either culture or PCR) for *B. breve*. However, 35% of the control infants were also colonised. By 36 weeks corrected gestational age, the infants within the experimental group had the same level of colonisation (84%) but nearly half of the control group (48.5%) had positive stool cultures [25]. Essentially, these data show that even the placebo group are being treated which would dilute the results and potentially cover up a beneficial effect. The mechanisms of colonisation for the control group, implicitly must be by 'cross-contamination' or rather spread between the infants within each unit. The results did show that the colonisation rates were higher in the smaller units. Smaller units are more likely to have participating infants close to each other.

Hygiene standards are very high in neonatal units because these infants are particularly vulnerable to sepsis. Despite this, an organism deliberately introduced was able to spread within the units. This makes designing high-quality studies very difficult. Randomised control trials rely on making as many factors as possible the same to avoid confounders. Valid data would not be generated if infants in the control group were not cared for in the same facilities as those receiving probiotics. The Cochrane review concludes that better quality studies are needed to answer this question properly but this is not straightforward. Whilst most studies did not collect this kind of data, it is inescapable that logically, all randomised studies of probiotics may be underestimating the beneficial effect because the control group is likely to be receiving treatment inadvertently. That is not the same thing as there being actual evidence of a benefit, of course.

The use of probiotics in preterm neonates to prevent NEC remains controversial. There is no clear evidence of a benefit overall. The data does suggest that they are safe but that has not completely relieved the concerns about potential sepsis. There is no clear consensus on which organism(s) should be given and because they are a food product rather than a medicine, the quality-control is not the same. For these reasons, it is very difficult to reach a conclusion about their use, which is disappointing as there had been hope that they could be a very effective measure for reducing the risk of NEC.

6.6 Infection Control

This is arguably an historical rather than a contemporary concern. In what could be considered the early days of NEC, there was a lot of focus on NEC as an infective disease. This reflects in part, that the role of microbial infection in NEC was emerging and also that NEC was seen to occur in clusters. In the modern age, for other reasons—i.e. preventing neonatal sepsis—infection control in a routine part of neonatology. It is very much assumed that basic infection control measures will be part of neonatal care. This explains why there is so little recent literature on infection control and NEC. It simply is not an active issue anymore. It is worth noting, of course, that the evidence from probiotic research shows that the biome of neonates cared for in the same unit can converge [25].

Stein et al. (1972) reported a series of 11 NEC cases in the same nursery over a 10 week period which is possibly the first report of a cluster or 'epidemic' of NEC [26]. Several similar clusters were reported subsequently and in some cases a responsible organism was identified. Work published over 30 years later suggest that NEC does still occur in clusters [27]. Whether such 'mini-epidemics' can be controlled and prevented is not clear.

Infection control is part of an NEC prevention strategy but there is no evidence that special measures over and above what would be considered standard practice in neonatology are necessary.

6.7 Preventing Necrotising Enterocolitis in Congenital Cardiac Disease

The incidence of NEC in full-term babies with congenital heart disease (CHD) is reported as somewhere between 1.6% and 6% [28]. Given that these babies are known to be specifically at risk and undergoing various medical and surgical interventions, there is undoubtedly a window of opportunity to enact measures to reduce the risk. Sadly, there is a paucity of evidence for any such measures that could be routinely used. To some extent this reflects the fact that whilst various risk factors are clearly known in this context, they are not easily modifiable ones.

6.7.1 Enteral Feeding

There is very limited evidence around feeding CHD infants after cardiac surgery but the data that does exists suggests that holding off enteral feeds and using parenteral nutrition does not reduce the risk of NEC. Infants fed early have shorter lengths of stay and avoid the risks associated with prolonged PN use [28, 29].

6.7.2 Association with Cardiac Surgery

It has been shown that NEC is more common during the postoperative period rather than prior to cardiac surgery [29]. This implies that the physiological insult of surgery is a greater risk (in terms of NEC) than the underlying cardiac lesion. That does not change the fact that infants with CHD are at risk of NEC untreated and that they need corrective surgery anyway. At present there is no detailed evidence to suggest an optimal timing of surgery to minimise the risk. This is somewhat inevitable as CHD is a multitude of very diverse conditions.

Conversely the window of highest risk is clearly defined (i.e. in the days following corrective surgery) and hence there is potential for the clinical application of any putative preventative interventions.

6.8 Future Prevention of NEC?

NEC remains a disease with poor outcomes and whilst treatment options are as limited as they are, the need for preventative strategies is all too clear. Chapter 10 discusses potential future therapies for NEC such as remote ischaemic conditioning. Remote conditioning could also be used preventatively if it is indeed effective in human neonates. In babies who have CHD there is a clear time-frame in which they are most at risk. Similarly, preterm babies born before 30 weeks completed gestation, develop NEC from the second week of life onwards. It would therefore be possible to institute measures to prevent NEC in these babies in these time-frames when they are most at risk.

References

1. Ohuma E, Moller A, Bradley E, Chakwera S, Hussain-Alkhateeb L, Lewin A, et al. National, regional, and global estimates of preterm birth in 2020, with trends from 2010: a systematic analysis. Lancet. 2023;402(10409):1261–71. https://doi.org/10.1016/S0140-6736(23)00878-4.
2. Perin J, Mulick A, Yeung D, Villavicencio F, Lopez G, Strong K, et al. Global, regional, and national causes of under-5 mortality in 2000–19: an updated systematic analysis with implications for the sustainable development goals. Lancet Child Adolesc Health. 2022;6(2):106–15. https://doi.org/10.1016/S2352-4642(21)00311-4.
3. NIH. Neonatal intensive care a history of excellence a symposium commemorating child health day. 1985. https://neonatology.net/pdf/nic.nih1985.pdf.
4. Newnham J, Dickinson J, Hart R, Pennell C, Arrese C, Keelan J. Strategies to prevent preterm birth. Front Immunol. 2014;5:756035. https://doi.org/10.3389/fimmu.2014.00584.
5. Dodd J, Jones L, Flenady V, Cincotta R, Crowther C. Prenatal administration of progesterone for preventing preterm birth in women considered to be at risk of preterm birth. Cochrane Database Syst Rev. 2013;7:CD004947. https://doi.org/10.1002/14651858.CD004947.pub3.
6. Smeenk J, Wyns C, De Geyter C, Kupka M, Bergh C, et al. ART in Europe, 2019: results generated from European registries by ESHRE†. Hum Reprod. 2023;38(12):2321–38. https://doi.org/10.1093/humrep/dead197.
7. Human Fertilisation and Embryology Authority. Fertility treatment 2021: preliminary trends and figures. HFEA. 2024. https://www.hfea.gov.uk/about-us/publications/research-and-data/fertility-treatment-2021-preliminary-trends-and-figures/#section-4.
8. Daskalakis G, Psarris A, Koutras A, Fasoulakis Z, Prokopakis I, Varthaliti A, et al. Maternal infection and preterm birth: from molecular basis to clinical implications. Children. 2023;10(5):907. https://doi.org/10.3390/children10050907.

9. Liggins G, Howie R. A controlled trial of antepartum glucocorticoid treatment for prevention of the respiratory distress syndrome in premature infants. Pediatrics. 1972;50(4):250–1.
10. Roberts D, Brown J, Medley N, Dalziel S. Antenatal corticosteroids for accelerating fetal lung maturation for women at risk of preterm birth. Cochrane Database Syst Rev. 2017;3(3):CD004454. https://doi.org/10.1002/14651858.CD004454.pub3.
11. Stock S, Thomson A, Papworth S, Royal College of Obstetricians and Gynaecologists. Antenatal corticosteroids to reduce neonatal morbidity and mortality: green-top guideline no. 74. BJOG. 2022;129(8):e35–60. https://doi.org/10.1111/1471-0528.17027.
12. Lu L, Lu J, Yu Y, Claud E. Necrotizing enterocolitis intestinal barrier function protection by antenatal dexamethasone and surfactant-D in a rat model. Pediatr Res. 2021;90(4):768–75. https://doi.org/10.1038/s41390-020-01334-0.
13. Berseth CL. Feeding strategies and necrotizing enterocolitis. Curr Opin Pediatr. 2005;17(2):170–3.
14. Sisk P, Lovelady C, Dillard R, Gruber K, O'Shea T. Early human milk feeding is associated with a lower risk of necrotizing enterocolitis in very low birth weight infants. J Perinatol. 2007;27(7):428–33. https://doi.org/10.1038/sj.jp.7211758.
15. Quigley MA, Henderson G, Anthony MY, McGuire W. Formula milk versus donor breast milk for feeding preterm or low birth weight infants. Cochrane Database Syst Rev. 2007;4:CD002971. https://doi.org/10.1002/14651858.CD002971.pub2.
16. Quigley M, McGuire W. Formula versus donor breast milk for feeding preterm or low birth weight infants. Cochrane Database Syst Rev. 2014;4:CD002971. https://doi.org/10.1002/14651858.CD002971.pub3.
17. Meinzen-Derr J, Poindexter B, Wrage L, Morrow A, Stoll B, Donovan E. Role of human milk in extremely low birth weight infants' risk of necrotizing enterocolitis or death. J Perinatol. 2009;29(1):57–62. https://doi.org/10.1038/jp.2008.117.
18. Embleton N, Jennifer MS, Lapillonne A, van den Akker C, Carnielli V, Fusch C, et al. Enteral Nutrition in Preterm Infants (2022): A Position Paper From the ESPGHAN Committee on Nutrition and Invited Experts. Journal of pediatric gastroenterology and nutrition. 2023;76(2). https://doi.org/10.1097/MPG.0000000000003642.
19. Morgan J, Young L, McGuire W. Slow advancement of enteral feed volumes to prevent necrotising enterocolitis in very low birth weight infants. Cochrane Database Syst Rev. 2011;3:CD001241. https://doi.org/10.1002/14651858.CD001241.pub3.
20. Oddie SJ, Young L, McGuire W. Slow advancement of enteral feed volumes to prevent necrotising enterocolitis in very low birth weight infants. Cochrane Database Syst Rev. 2017;8:CD001241. https://doi.org/10.1002/14651858.CD001241.pub7.
21. Dorling J, Abbott J, Berrington J, Bosiak B, Bowler U, Boyle E, et al. Controlled trial of two incremental milk-feeding rates in preterm infants. N Engl J Med. 2019;381(15):1434–43. https://doi.org/10.1056/NEJMoa1816654.
22. Sharif S, Meader N, Oddie S, Rojas-Reyes M, McGuire W. Probiotics to prevent necrotising enterocolitis in very preterm or very low birth weight infants. Cochrane Database Syst Rev. 2023;7(7):CD005496. https://doi.org/10.1002/14651858.CD005496.pub6.
23. Lewis Z, Shani G, Masarweh C, Popovic M, Frese S, Sela D, et al. Validating bifidobacterial species and subspecies identity in commercial probiotic products. Pediatr Res. 2016;79(3):445–52. https://doi.org/10.1038/pr.2015.244.
24. Costeloe K, Hardy P, Juszczak E, Wilks M, Millar M. Bifidobacterium breve BBG-001 in very preterm infants: a randomised controlled phase 3 trial. Lancet. 2016;387(10019):649–60. https://doi.org/10.1016/S0140-6736(15)01027-2.
25. Costeloe K, Bowler U, Brocklehurst P, Hardy P, Heal P, Juszczak E, et al. A randomised controlled trial of the probiotic bifidobacterium breve BBG-001 in preterm babies to prevent sepsis, necrotising enterocolitis and death: the probiotics in preterm infants (PiPS) trial. Health Technol Assess. 2016;20(66):1–194. https://doi.org/10.3310/hta20660.
26. Stein H, Beck J, Solomon A, Schmaman A. Gastroenteritis with necrotizing enterocolitis in premature babies. Br Med J. 1972;2(5814):616–9. https://doi.org/10.1136/bmj.2.5814.616.

27. Meinzen-Derr J, Morrow A, Hornung R, Donovan E, Dietrich K, Succop P. Epidemiology of necrotizing enterocolitis temporal clustering in two neonatology practices. J Pediatr. 2009;154(5):656–61. https://doi.org/10.1016/j.jpeds.2008.11.002.
28. Kashif H, Abuelgasim E, Hussain N, Luyt J, Harky A. Necrotizing enterocolitis and congenital heart disease. Ann Pediatr Cardiol. 2021;14(4):539–52. https://doi.org/10.4103/apc.apc_30_21.
29. Nordenström K, Lannering K, Mellander M, Elfvin A. Low risk of necrotising enterocolitis in enterally fed neonates with critical heart disease: an observational study. Arch Dis Child Fetal Neonatal Ed. 2020;105(6):609–14. https://doi.org/10.1136/archdischild-2019-318537.

Chapter 7
Clinical Management of Necrotising Enterocolitis

Contents

Abstract Necrotising enterocolitis is a clinical diagnosis. The presenting history, examination findings and investigations are all important in making the diagnosis of NEC. In clinical practice many babies with early disease (Bell stage I or equivalent) may be indistinguishable from other diagnoses in preterm infants. These babies should be treated as NEC and reviewed after 48 h when the diagnosis often becomes clearer. Babies with confirmed NEC require medical management for a period of 7–10 days and may require surgery.

Babies with NEC will typically have systemic upset, abdominal distension and bilious aspirates. They may have blood in their stools. In the presence of such symptoms, pneumotosis intestinalis on x-ray or ultrasound scan confirms the diagnosis.

© The Author(s), under exclusive license to Springer Nature Switzerland AG 2024

I. Jones, *Necrotising Enterocolitis in Clinical Practice*, In Clinical Practice, https://doi.org/10.1007/978-3-031-64148-0_7

Medical treatment for NEC remains supportive only with babies receiving gut rest and decompression and broad-spectrum antibiotics. Some infants will develop multi-organ failure and require ventilatory and cardiovascular support.

Babies who are successfully treated for NEC may go on to develop intestinal strictures.

Keywords NEC treatment options · NEC management protocols · Medical management of NEC · Surgical management of NEC · Bell's staging criteria for NEC · Antibiotic therapy for NEC · Bowel rest in NEC management · Enteral feeding strategies in NEC · Parenteral nutrition in NEC management · Monitoring for NEC complications · Fluid management in NEC · Hemodynamic support in NEC · Respiratory support in NEC · Pain management in NEC · Nutrition support in NEC · Surgical indications for NEC · Timing of surgical intervention in NEC Surgical techniques for NEC · Postoperative care in NEC · Long-term follow-up in NEC survivors

7.1   Introduction

The focus of this chapter is the diagnosis and medical management of NEC. Surgery for NEC is discussed fully in the next chapter. Whilst this is a slightly false separation, it does allow space for a full discussion on the issues around when to operate and surgical strategies for NEC.

NEC is both a medical and surgical disease. The majority of babies with a diagnosis of NEC do not undergo surgery. It is undoubtedly true that many of the babies who meet the criteria for Bell Stage I do not in fact have NEC. The initial features are very nonspecific. In practice, babies that undergo surgery have most often had a period of 'medical management' first before clinical deterioration leads to a need for more invasive intervention. It is rare that babies with NEC present with a pneumoperitoneum due to perforation initially. NEC tends to be a progressive disease over hours or days.

The chapter ends with two case studies designed to illustrate the points in practice.

7.2   Diagnosis

NEC remains a clinical diagnosis with no single test including or excluding the diagnosis. Hence, the classical approach of history, examination and investigations taken together allow the formation of a diagnosis.

7.2.1   History

The typical history of NEC is a premature baby that is more than a week of age and has been established on enteral feeds. The baby develops abdominal distension, vomiting and/or increased gastric aspirates from the nasogastric (or orogastric) tube. These aspirates tend to be bilious. Stooling stops or they pass blood in their stool. The babies often become lethargic.

7.2.2   Examination and Clinical Signs

The first clinical sign is usually abdominal distension (Fig. 7.1). Other signs include temperature instability, irritability, bradycardia, apnoea and haemodynamic compromise. These collectively are signs of sepsis which is the key differential diagnosis. Most often this is sepsis from a non-abdominal cause with a secondary septic ileus causing the abdominal signs. It is often the case that these two diagnoses are indistinguishable at an early stages. Moreover, it is not always possible to tell the difference retrospectively.

As the disease progresses, the abdominal signs may become more pronounced. Perforation is often accompanied by marked discolouration of the skin. In the early stages, the abdomen is distended but soft. In more advanced disease the abdomen can become hard and there can be demonstrable tenderness. Sometimes a mass is palpable. Abdominal wall oedema and erythema are often seen.

Abdominal signs can be subtle in premature neonates and experience at examining neonates is invaluable in eliciting clinical signs. Abdominal tenderness may be evident in observed pain responses such as changes in facial expression. Tenderness can also be demonstrated by an infant that becomes bradycardic, bradypnoeic and desaturates on examination. In the most premature babies, the abdominal wall musculature is very underdeveloped as therefore true guarding is much less obvious than in an adult or older child.

Fig. 7.1 Abdominal distension in a neonate

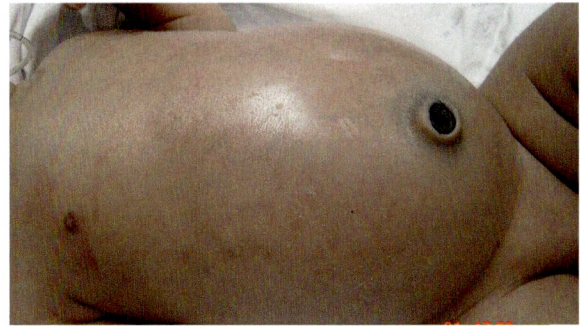

7.2.3   Investigations

Any infant with suspected NEC needs blood tests and an abdominal radiograph. A venous blood gas may also be indicated.

7.2.3.1   Blood Tests

The blood test results seen in NEC are mostly non-specific and indicate an inflammatory process. A standard assessment would include a full blood count, creatinine, urea and electrolytes, glucose and C-reactive protein (CRP).

The white cell count can be raised or indeed low, in keeping with sepsis. C-reactive protein is a non-specific opsonin and a classical acute-phase reactant. It is often raised early in sepsis and may be high whilst the full blood count is normal. In babies, any rise in CRP is noteworthy. These babies also often have blood glucose instability and in more severe disease, electrolyte upset is seen.

Thrombocytopenia is arguably the most important laboratory finding in NEC. A drop in the platelet count is part of the diagnosis but it has also been shown to be prognostic; both in terms of the likelihood of needing surgery and mortality [1].

Metabolic acidosis and a raised lactate are also features of NEC. Again these are non-specific findings and are compatible with other causes of sepsis.

7.2.3.2   Radiological Findings

Figure 7.2 shows a classical NEC abdominal x-ray with pneumatosis intestinalis. Pneumotosis is a 'bubby' appearance seen on the abdominal film which indicates gas within the intestinal wall. Stool residue in the intestine has a similar appearance and distinguishing pneumotosis from stool residue is sometimes difficult. The position of the 'bubbles' can be a useful discriminator as stool residue is only seen in the colon.

It should be noted, however, that many babies with NEC do not have such clear-cut, diagnostic features – especially in the early stages of the disease. It is much more common for babies with NEC to initially have non-specific findings on an abdominal film. Typically these patients will have multiple visible bowel loops with increased spacing between the gas-filled lumens on plain x-ray. This finding is often described as a 'thickened bowel wall appearance.' This description is not strictly correct as the same appearance is seen with free fluid in the abdomen. Hence, a more precise description is to describe this increased spacing between the gas-filled intestinal lumens. This is not critical from a pragmatic point of view, as either way, both the presence of a thickened bowel wall due to inflammation and free fluid in the abdomen (also due to intra-abdominal inflammation) are consistent with NEC. They remain however, non-specific findings as they are consistent with other pathologies.

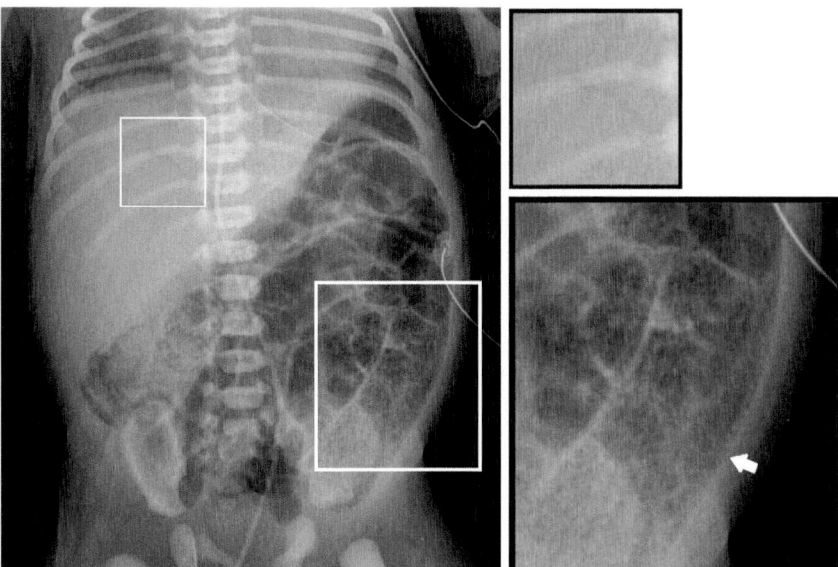

Fig. 7.2 Abdominal radiograph of necrotising enterocolitis This image shows a nasogastric in the stomach and a umbilical venous catheter. There is extensive pneumotosis, in both the right lower and left lower quadrant. In the left lower quadrant there may also be 'tram-lining' [Insert, arrow] There is portal venous gas [insert]

In the context of a baby with the clinical features of NEC, the presence of gas within the intestinal wall is considered pathopneumonic for NEC. The presence of gas within in the bowel wall due to the invasion of gas-forming bacteria. This was established by detailed analysis of the gas itself. In the same experiment, both luminal and mural gas was sampled in surgical specimens. This contained more than 30% hydrogen. Nitrogen, carbon dioxide and traces of oxygen were also found. Hydrogen is not found in ambient air and is not a product of human metabolism, implying a bacterial source. Bacteria taken from the same patients were cultured and they produced hydrogen gas. Intriguingly in these experiments, the bacteria only produced hydrogen when given a substrate of milk or 50% glucose [2]. The gas can also track from the intestinal wall into the portal venous system and be visible on a plain x-ray. Figure 7.2 shows both extensive pneumotosis, especially in the left lower quadrant and gas in the portal venous system. There is also pneumotosis on the right side. The left side in highlighted in the insert where the arrow indicates 'tram-lining' where the gas bubbles are visible in a line showing a separation between the layers of the intestinal wall. This is thought to correspond to deeper invasion. The gas (and therefore presumably the bacteria) is initially found in the submucosal layer but progresses to be transmural. Pneumotosis is also a transient radiological sign. It may be present on an abdominal x-ray and then absent a few hours later.

Soni et al. [3] published a very good review of radiological findings in NEC with excellent examples of the kind of appearance that is most often seen but to summarise:

1. Most babies with NEC will have non-specific findings on abdominal radiograph i.e. dilated intestinal bowel loops, separation between the gas-filled lumen
2. The presence of pneumotosis is diagnostic in a baby with clinical signs and symptoms of NEC
3. It is important to look for signs of perforation or other indications for surgery

7.2.4 Making the Diagnosis

The (modified) Bell classification for NEC is the most widely-used diagnostic criteria for NEC [4]. The modified Bell classification is summarised in Table 3.1, in the chapter on the definition of NEC. There are two key points here for clinical management of NEC. The onset of NEC can be insidious and the clinical features consistent with other diagnoses. NEC can also progress to fulminant disease rapidly. Therefore any baby with suspected NEC requires close monitoring and repeated assessment.

From a clinical perspective, the differential between Bell stage I and II is of limited relevance initially. Whilst many babies who fit the definition for Bell stage I will not have NEC, the initial treatment is the same: they should all be treated as NEC. The other diagnostic criteria mentioned in Chap. 3 are arguably more robust but the initial supportive management is the same.

7.3 Medical Therapy

Initial management of NEC is very simple. It involves withholding feeds and providing decompression of the stomach and intestines with a nasogastric (or orogastric) tube. Parenteral nutrition should also be given. Broad spectrum antibiotics should be started and organ support given as needed. There will be some inevitable variation in practice as the diagnosis is still dependent on clinical judgement. However a typical regime would be to treat all babies who meet the criteria for Bell stage I with 48 h of antibiotics, gut rest and decompression before reassessing. Some of these infants will recover and can be safely fed at this point. Others will at this point (or earlier) meet the criteria for Bell stage II and therefore should be treated for 7–10 days. Surveys show that practice does vary quite lot. One such protocol advocates treating babies with Bell Stage I for 48 h, IIa for 7 days, IIb and IIIa for 10 days and IIIb for 14 days [5].

Over the years, there has been considerable interest in biomarkers as diagnostic and prognostic tools in NEC. At the time of writing there is no consensus to support the routine use of any such tests in the clinical decision-making around NEC management. However, the following have all been considered: CRP, intestinal fatty acid binding protein (i-FABP), interleukin-6, lactate, Serum Ameloid A. The potential role in prognostication, especially distinguishing medical and surgical disease is discussed in Sect. 8.1.4.

7.3.1 Antibiotics

A systematic review concluded that "[in]sufficient evidence was found for any recommendation on the choice of antibiotics, the route of administration or the duration in infants treated for NEC" [6]. Four out of five of the included studies in this review are from the 1980s.

Babies with NEC should receive broad-spectrum antibiotics. It may be the case that including metronidazole in the regimen to cover intestinal anaerobic organisms is important but the data is not sufficient to state this with confidence [6].

7.3.2 Cessation of Enteral Feeds

The role of enteral feeding in the pathogenesis of NEC is well-established. Historically, evidence suggested that rapid increases in feeds or larger feed volumes were associated with NEC [7]. Which is why the withholding of feeds is so embedded in NEC treatment. Data from the 1970s suggested that re-introducing feeds before 10 days was associated with 'disease recurrence' in many patients [8].

Neonatal care has evolved a lot since then and the use of feeding regimens protocols is now standard practice. The SIFT trial demonstrated that more rapid advancing of feeds from birth can be done safely [9]. Notwithstanding this result, the data is clear that enteral feeding is a key trigger for NEC and removing this stimulus is therefore logical. This pathophysiology unquestionably implies that cessation of feeding has to be part of NEC management. What is much less clear is how long, infants with NEC should have their feeds withheld. There is very limited evidence on how long feeding should be withheld and significant variation in practice [10]. Most practitioners would consider reintroducing feeds after 48 h in an infant with Bell stage I (suspected NEC), if they recover and do not go on to Bell stage II. With a clear diagnosis of NEC (IIa or above) then 7–10 days of treatment is commonplace.

There is some evidence that feeds can be reintroduced earlier although it is understandable that in practice a more conservative approach is taken whilst the evidence remains limited.

One study, from the early 2000s used a protocol of re-introducing feeds from 3 days, if the patient was well and there was no evidence of portal venous gas on ultrasound scan [10]. By using this approach, the median time to reintroduction of feeds after a diagnosis of NEC was 4 days, compared to 10 days in the historical control group. This was associated with a shorter time to full feeds, a shorter length of stay and a lower rate of central-venous catheter-related sepsis. The significance of portal venous gas as a marker for disease severity in NEC has long been debated [11], and it is not entirely clear why this marker was chosen here. However it does highlight that there are negative sequelae of withholding feeds and/or giving antibiotics for a prolonged period. The risk of recurrent or progressive disease needs to be balanced against the consequences of withholding feeds.

Kuik et al. (2020) looked at markers of intestinal recovery to see if there was a method for guiding the reintroduction of feeds. They measured regional intestinal oxygen saturation ($r_{int}SO_2$) by means of near-infrared spectrometry and serum intestinal-fatty acid binding protein (iFABP) [12]. They showed that $r_{int}SO_2$ levels are a good predictor of intestinal recovery but only after the intestine is exposed to feeding once again. Hence, it could only be used to guide advancement of feeding, not to determine when to restart feed.

This is an area where NEC practice is essentially historical and there is a paucity of evidence as to what might be best practice. Disease severity it likely to be important: milder forms of the disease would probably allow earlier feeding whilst in more severe cases, a more prolonged pause in feeding may well be necessary to prevent disease progression. Chap. 10 focuses on novel treatments of NEC but there is also significant scope for research to optimise current therapy. Both basic science research and clinical trials are needed. A biomarker that allowed individual decision-making about the length of treatment would make a big difference to clinical practice. Similarly, clear data on the risks and benefits of timing of feed reintroduction does not currently exist.

In summary, all babies with NEC need to have feeds withheld for a period of time. Local protocols vary but the majority of centres will treat Bell stage I for 48 h and Bell stage II for between 5 and10 days. Some protocols advocate up to 14 days for Bell stage III.

7.4   Multi-Organ Failure and Organ Support

Multi-organ failure is a feature of severe NEC. In essence, management of multi-organ failure in NEC is no different from intensive care management of patients with any other diagnosis. These babies often need mechanical ventilation and inotropic support. Ventilator strategies in premature babies are vitally important for reducing the risk of lung injury. Lung immaturity is the major contributor to long-term respiratory morbidity but ventilator-induced lung injury is also a key factor [13]. In the most unwell infants, high-frequency oscillatory ventilation (HFOV) is often needed to reduce the risk of barotrauma. This is not uncommon in the most unwell infants with NEC.

Low systemic blood flow is common in extremely premature (less than 30 weeks gestation) infants from multiple causes. It is associated with brain injury, developmental impairment and death. The same inotropic agents used in other patient groups are used in premature neonates. However there is a paucity of evidence as to which agents might be preferable and confer a better outcome. A Cochrane review concluded that there is limited evidence that dobutamine may be better than dopamine at increasing and maintaining systemic blood flow [14].

A recent review further highlighted the lack of evidence in the management of hypotension in preterm babies and argues that an over-reliance on mean blood pressure (MAP) means that therapy is not optimised [15]. This is important because cardiac physiology is known to be different in premature babies and the distribution of the relevant receptors that these agents act on is also not the same as in term infants. They argue that simply targeting MAP, whilst simple and straight-forward, is the wrong approach for preterm babies.

In the context of NEC (and sepsis) where a 'warm-shock' develops, these babies will initially have a high heart rate, a normal systolic pressure but a low diastolic blood pressure. At this point, vasopressive agents such as noradrenaline (norepinephrine) may be the most effective but myocardial contractility can deteriorate and result in 'cold-shock' as increased systemic resistance is the physiological response designed to divert blood flow to essential organs. At this point, agents that increase myocardial contractility are needed such as adrenaline (epinephrine). Corticosteroids may also be important as most of these babies have effective adrenal insufficiency [15]. The choice of agent also has an impact on disease progression. Vasopressive agents reduce blood flow to the intestine which may make NEC worse and most surgeons would not consider an anastomosis following bowel resection whilst the infant is receiving them.

7.5   Surgery for NEC?

Currently, routine practice in NEC is to treat it medically *unless and until* there is an indication for surgery. The indications for surgery and the debate about timing of surgery are discussed in detail in the next chapter. Most infants with NEC (between 50% and 70%) do not have acute surgery [16, 17]. Therefore, in the majority of cases, NEC is a disease managed medically by neonatologists.

7.6   Post NEC Intestinal Strictures

Following successful medical management of NEC, a proportion of infants will develop intestinal strictures. The majority of strictures are seen between the fourth and eighth week after the acute episode of NEC [18].

Classically, these infants tend to have recurrent episodes of feed intolerance with advancing feeds. A typical history would be an infant without signs of sepsis but with abdominal distension and raised gastric aspirates. The aspirates are typically bilious. It's not unusual for these babies to tolerate a small volume of feed but advancement of feeds results in distension and vomiting. A post NEC stricture should be suspected in an infant with evidence of obstruction and a history of an episode of NEC.

Contrast radiology is the most common diagnostic test. Barium can be used or a water-soluable contrast agent. The majority of strictures occur in the colon. Small bowel strictures are most commly seen in the distal small bowel [18]. For this reason, a lower GI contrast study is more likely to be useful and is usually performed first. If this is not diagnostic, an upper GI contrast study and follow-through (with delayed film(s)) may delineate the stricture. If the upper GI study is performed first, the lack of clearance of contrast medium makes performing a subsequent lower study technically challenging. The residue contrast prevents clear delineation of the intestine.

Intestinal strictures require surgical resection but as these babies are normally not unwell, apart from their feed intolerance, it is generally much lower risk surgery. These infants usually tolerate the anaesthetic and surgery very well and a primary anastomosis in normally performed.

7.7   Ethical Considerations

It would be inappropriate for a volume on NEC not to include some consideration of the ethical and moral challenges that are unavoidable when caring for these babies. NEC is devastating disease and often the biggest challenge for clinicians and families is dealing with decision-making when the prognosis may not be known with any great certainty and increasingly invasive treatments are being considered.

In the UK, in 2006, the Nuffield Council on Bioethics published a thorough and wide-ranging report on critical care decisions in foetal and neonatal medicine with detailed recommendations on best practice [19]. The working party that produced the report included neonatologists, an obstetrician, a children's nursing professor, philosophers, social scientists, lawyers, a health economist, and individuals who have worked with families of extremely premature babies and disabled children. The report is to some extent out of date now as the recommendations for initial management of babies born at 22 and 23 weeks gestation have been superseded. Advancements in care have changed the prognosis for these babies and accordingly, guidelines have changed [20]. However, the Nuffield report is thorough and wide-ranging and the principals outlined for clinical decision-making remain relevant and crucial. Indeed the change in practice at the extreme of viability is not because the ethical framework has changed but because outcomes have improved.

The report explores the key concept that clinicians are required to always act in the best interests of the patient, which may involve a decision to withhold or withdraw active treatment.

> After an initial decision has been taken to start intensive care, there may come a time when parents and doctors begin discussing whether withdrawing active treatment would be in the best interests of the baby.

It goes on to say that the reasons for withdrawing care, generally fit one of the following three groups: (1) When intensive care is futile, and death appears inevitable; (2) When a baby has suffered a severe brain injury and for whom there appears to a very high risk of severe disability; and (3) When a baby is discovered to have a serious malformation for which there is no treatment.

In the specific context of NEC, all three of these can apply. In some babies clinical teams may feel that a laparotomy is futile as the physiological state of the baby is sufficiently dire that they will not survive surgery. A baby who undergoes surgery and is found to have *nec totalis* where the entire small bowel is necrotic pose a particular challenge as theoretically a complete resection can be done but this commits the infant to long-term PN and potentially small bowel transplant years later. Both of which are significantly morbid.

It is important to look at the overall status of the infant. Brain injury in the form of intraventricular haemorrhage (IVH) or periventricular leukomalacia (PVL) may be demonstrated by cranial ultrasound (Sect. 9.4.3). A baby with a mild grade of IVH may well develop more severe IVH following an episode of NEC conferring a poor neurological outcome.

The primary focus of care is, of course, one of active treatment with an intention to manage the acute episode and prevent long-term consequences. However, it remains the case that for some of these babies, palliative treatments which concentrate on minimising pain and distress will be needed.

7.8 Case Studies

7.8.1 Case Study 1

This case concerns a baby boy born at 26 weeks and 2 days gestation. It was a spontaneous labour with prolonged rupture of membranes, around 72 h prior to delivery and the mother received antenatal corticosteroids prior to delivery. He was 645 g at birth.

He has had non-invasive ventilatory support only and is now 15 days old. He was advanced on feeds as per protocol, and reached full feeds which he was tolerating well. He was only fed with maternal breast milk until 2 days ago when a cows-milk based fortifier was added due to faltering growth.

In the last 12 h he has developed abdominal distension and has green aspirates from his orogastric tube. These aspirates are measured every 3 h and have been 12, 18, 20 and 22 mL respectively.

Q1.What features are important for clinical assessment?

A1: *A global examination of the baby's status is critical. Review of respiratory status includes whether he has developed an oxygen requirement but also whether he is having apnoeas and/or brachycardic episodes. Abdominal examination will include any changes of skin colour as well as an assessment for signs of peritonism. Review of the bedside chart includes the record of stooling and whether there was any blood in the stool.*

In this case, he has been started on oxygen at 0.2 L/min flow via nasal cannula but has not had any apnoeic episodes. His pulse and blood pressure are within the normal range for gestational age. Abdominal examination reveals gaseous distension of the abdomen with no discolouration. He demonstrates no tenderness and he tolerated being examined well. He has not stooled for 24 h.

Q2. What investigations should be performed at this stage.

A2: *Venous blood should be taken for a full blood count, urea, creatinine and electrolytes and C-reactive protein and blood cultures. Liver-function tests may be useful to assess the bilirubin level. A venous blood gas may be useful. A plain abdominal x-ray should be taken looking for specific signs of NEC.*

The blood tests and abdominal x-ray report are shown here:

Full Blood Count			Abdominal X-ray Report
Haemoglobin	152 g/l	(134-199)	
Haematocrit	0.51 l/l	(0.32-0.65)	Anterio-posterior abdominal x-ray dated
White Cell Count	10.0×10^9/l	(6.0-21.0)	*[today]* shows a non-specific bowel gas
Platelets	152×10^9/l	(150-450)	pattern. There are multiple loops of small
Differential White Cell Count:			bowel with mild to moderate distension.
Neutrophils	7.0×10^9/l	(1.5-5.4)	There is no visible gas in the rectum.
Lymphocytes	2.4×10^9/l	(2.8-9.1)	
Monocytes	0.3×10^9/l	(0.1-1.7)	No pneumotosis of portal-venous gas is seen
			on this film and there is no evidence of free
Biochemistry			gas.
Creatinine	22 mmol/l	(16-47)	
Urea	7.1 mmol/l	(1.1-8.0)	
Sodium	142 mmol/l	(136-146)	
Potassium	4.1 mmol/l	(3.5-5.3)	
C-reactive protein	14 mg/l	(<5.0)	
References ranges vary by laboratory			

Q3. What management should be instituted at this point?

A3: *This baby has some clear risk factors for NEC. He born prematurely and was small for his gestation age. Whether fortifiers are a true risk factor for NEC remains controversial. He did receive antenatal corticosteroids, which is known to provide some protection. The blood tests are unremarkable apart from a small rise in CRP. The abdominal x-ray is consistent with NEC but not diagnostic. Currently he has all the features of Bell stage I NEC (see Table 3.1) and therefore management at this stage would include: Stopping enteral feeds, placing the orogastric tube on free drainage (and/or regular aspiration) for gastric decompression, the* *commencement of broad-spectrum IV antibiotics and regular review of the baby's progress. Parenteral nutrition should be given.*

The baby is closely monitored for 48 h. His abdominal distension resolves, he stools normally without blood and his aspirates become clear and of minimal volume. The blood cultures were negative. His CRP is now 3 mg/L.

Q4. What management is appropriate at this stage?

Given that he has recovered fully and never met the criteria for Bell stage II or above, antibiotics can be stopped and feeds restarted.

7.8.2 Case Study 2

A 12 day old baby girl was born at 35 weeks gestation with a birthweight of 2430 g. Antenally, she was diagnosed with a complex cardiac lesion and so delivery was planned in a specialist cardiac centre. She has a complex cardiac lesion that results in a low-output state but the multi-disciplinary decision is that she does not require cardiac surgery in the neonatal period. She has remained ventilated and has had continuous enteral feeds via an NG tube. Her formula feeds have been gradually advanced and she is currently receiving around 60 mL/kg of enteral feed in 24 h. Now in the second week of life, she is on minimal ventilator settings and all inotropic support has been stopped. She remains on diuretics.

At this point she develops abdominal distension and visible blood is seen in her stools. Clinical assessment reveals that she is cardiovascularly stable with a distended but soft abdomen. There is no obvious discolouration of the abdomen. Her blood tests are unremarkable. An abdominal x-ray is taken (Fig. 7.3).

Q1. Describe the findings on the abdominal radiograph

A1: *This film is slightly rotated but is a technically adequate film. There is a nasogastric tube within the stomach. The cardiac shadow shows an enlarged heart. There is an abnormal abdominal gas pattern with prominent bowel loops in the right and mid abdomen. In the right iliac fossa there is increased spacing between the gas-filled lumen consistent with thickening of the intestinal wall or free fluid. There is a paucity of gas in the pelvis. There is no pneumotosis or portal venous gas on this film. No free gas is identified.*

As she clearly meets the criteria for NEC Bell stage Ib, treatment is initiated with broad spectrum intravenous antibiotics and enteral feeds are paused. Parenteral nutrition is increased to 100% of her nutritional requirement.

She is regularly reviewed and 24 h later, the clinical picture is similar. Repeated blood tests are unremarkable, she has not required inotropic support. Ventilatory settings have increased slightly and the abdominal examination is the same, with a soft, distended abdomen and no discolouration or tenderness. A repeat abdominal film is taken which is shown below (Fig. 7.4):

Fig. 7.3 Case Study 2
abdominal radiograph

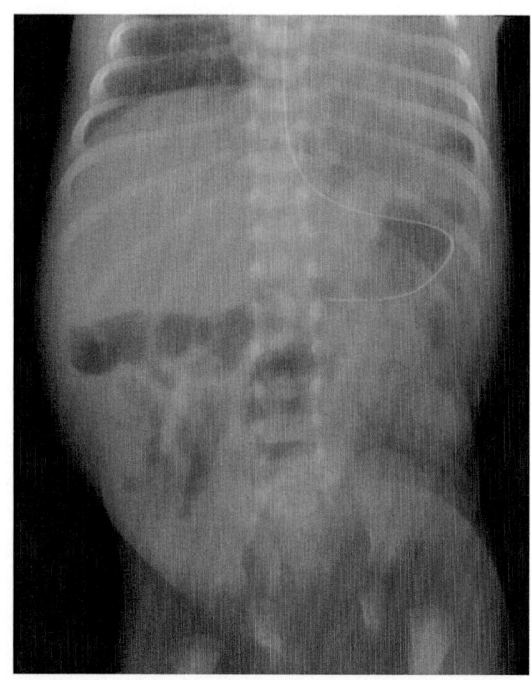

Fig. 7.4 Case Study 2
abdominal radiograph

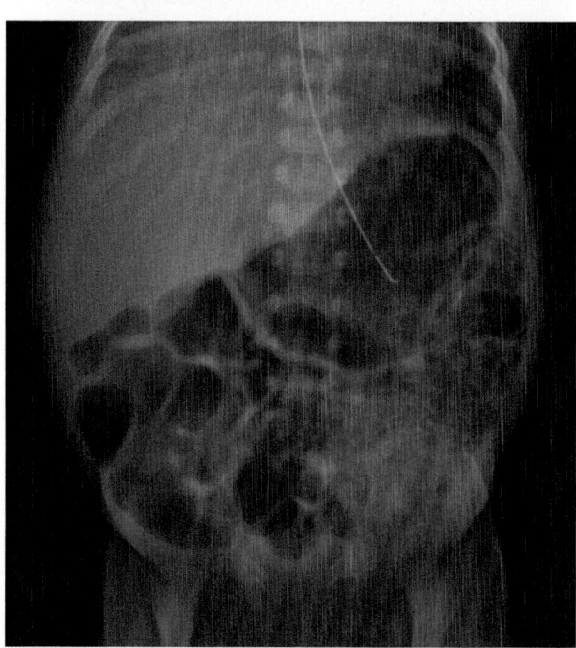

Q2. What does this radiograph show and does this change the management of this baby?

A2. *The gas pattern has changed significantly since the previous x-ray. There is now clear pneumotosis intestinalis in the left iliac fossa which is quite extensive. Portal venous gas is not demonstrated and there is no evidence of free gas.*

This baby now meets the criteria for Bell stage II and has confirmed NEC. The current management is the same: intravenous antibiotics, withholding of enteral feeds and gastric decompression. However, the option of stopping antibiotics at 48 h is now not appropriate and a prolonged course of treatment (typically 7 days) with careful review is indicated. At present there is no indication for surgery but close monitoring is mandated for the next 48–72 h at least.

References

1. Ragazzi S, Pierro A, Peters M, Fasoli L, Eaton S. Early full blood count and severity of disease in neonates with necrotizing enterocolitis. Pediatr Surg Int. 2003;19(5):376–9. https://doi.org/10.1007/s00383-003-1014-5.
2. Engel RR, Virning NL, Hunt CE. Origin of mural gas in necrotizing enterocolitis. Pediatr Res. 1973;7:292.
3. Soni R, Katana A, Curry JI, Humphries PD, Huertas-Ceballos A. How to use abdominal X-rays in preterm infants suspected of developing necrotising enterocolitis. Arch Dis Child Educ Pract Ed. 2020;105(1):50–7.
4. Patel R, Ferguson J, McElroy S, Khashu M, Caplan M. Defining necrotizing enterocolitis: current difficulties and future opportunities. Pediatr Res. 2020;88(Suppl 1):10–5. https://doi.org/10.1038/s41390-020-1074-4.
5. Aurora M, Keyes M, Acosta J, Swartz K, Lombay J, Ciaramitaro J, et al. Standardizing the evaluation and management of necrotizing enterocolitis in a level IV NICU. Pediatrics. 2022;150(4):e2022056616. https://doi.org/10.1542/peds.2022-056616.
6. Gill E, Jung K, Qvist N, Ellebæk M. Antibiotics in the medical and surgical treatment of necrotizing enterocolitis. A systematic review. BMC Pediatr. 2022;22(1):66. https://doi.org/10.1186/s12887-022-03120-9.
7. Goldman H. Feeding and necrotizing enterocolitis. Am J Dis Child (1960). 1980;134(6):553–5. https://doi.org/10.1001/archpedi.1980.02130180011004.
8. Frantz I, L'heureux P, Engel R, Hunt C. Necrotizing enterocolitis. J Pediatr. 1975;86(2):259–63. https://doi.org/10.1016/s0022-3476(75)80485-9.
9. Dorling J, Abbott J, Berrington J, Bosiak B, Bowler U, Boyle E, et al. Controlled trial of two incremental milk-feeding rates in preterm infants. N Engl J Med. 2019;381(15):1434–43. https://doi.org/10.1056/NEJMoa1816654.
10. Bohnhors TB, Müller S, Dördelmann M, Peter C, Petersen C, Poets C. Early feeding after necrotizing enterocolitis in preterm infants. J Pediatr. 2003;143(4):484–7. https://doi.org/10.1067/S0022-3476(03)00443-8.
11. Buras R, Guzzetta P, Avery G, Naulty C. Acidosis and hepatic portal venous gas: indications for surgery in necrotizing enterocolitis. Pediatrics. 1986;78(2):273–7.
12. Kuik S, Kalteren W, Mebius M, Bos A, Hulscher J, Kooi E. Predicting intestinal recovery after necrotizing enterocolitis in preterm infants. Pediatr Res. 2020;87(5):903–9. https://doi.org/10.1038/s41390-019-0634-y.
13. Chen I, Chen H. New developments in neonatal respiratory management. Pediatr Neonatol. 2022;63(4):341–7. https://doi.org/10.1016/j.pedneo.2022.02.002.

14. Osborn D, Paradisis M, Evans N. The effect of inotropes on morbidity and mortality in preterm infants with low systemic or organ blood flow. Cochrane Database Syst Rev. 2007;2007(1):CD005090. https://doi.org/10.1002/14651858.CD005090.pub2.
15. Mullaly R, El-Khuffash A. Haemodynamic assessment and management of hypotension in the preterm. Arch Dis Child Fetal Neonatal Ed. 2024;109(2):120–7. https://doi.org/10.1136/archdischild-2022-324935.
16. Allin B, Long AM, Gupta A, Knight M, Lakhoo K. A UK wide cohort study describing management and outcomes for infants with surgical Necrotising Enterocolitis. Sci Rep. 2017;7:41149. https://doi.org/10.1038/srep41149.
17. Liu Y, Qiao L, Wu X, Jiang Z, Hao X. Predictive factors for the surgical treatment of necrotizing enterocolitis in preterm infants: a single-center retrospective study. BMC Pediatr. 2022;22(1):9. https://doi.org/10.1186/s12887-021-02973-w.
18. Liu W, Wang Y, Zhu J, Zhang C, Liu G, Wang X, et al. Clinical features and management of post-necrotizing enterocolitis strictures in infants: a multicentre retrospective study. Medicine. 2020;99(19):e20209. https://doi.org/10.1097/MD.0000000000020209.
19. Nuffield Council on Bioethics. Critical care decisions in fetal and neonatal medicine: ethical issues. London: Nuffield Council on Bioethics; 2006.
20. Mahase E. Consider active management for premature babies born at 22 weeks, says new guidance. BMJ. 2019;367:l6151. https://doi.org/10.1136/bmj.l6151.

Chapter 8
Surgical Management of Necrotising Enterocolitis

Contents

Abstract Between 20% and 40% of infants with NEC will require surgical treatment. The absolute indication for surgery is radiological evidence of intestinal perforation. In the absence of this, it can be very challenging to identify clearly which infants need surgical intervention. Multiple other factors have been identified that suggest the need for surgery but currently there is no single factor that allows simple discrimination between those that will recover with medical therapy alone and those

I. Jones, *Necrotising Enterocolitis in Clinical Practice*, In Clinical Practice,
https://doi.org/10.1007/978-3-031-64148-0_8

that need intervention. There is good evidence that, with appropriate experience, abdominal ultrasonography is effective but it remains operator dependent.

There is undoubtedly a role for peritoneal drainage as a stabilising procedure for NEC with perforation, in infants who cannot tolerate a laparotomy and potentially as a definitive intervention.

Some babies who have intestinal resection will need a stoma but in the majority of cases, primary anastomosis is a safe and effective option. There is also a role for laparostomy and a 'second-look' procedure in the surgical management of NEC.

Keywords Surgical management of NEC · NEC surgical intervention · Surgical treatment for NEC · Necrotising Enterocolitis surgery · Surgical indications for NEC · Timing of surgical intervention in NEC · NEC surgical techniques Surgical options for NEC · Emergency surgery for NEC · Bowel resection in NEC Perforation repair in NEC · Ostomy creation in NEC · NEC surgical complications Postoperative care in NEC surgery · Long-term outcomes of NEC surgery Surgical consultation for NEC · Multidisciplinary approach to NEC surgery Laparoscopic surgery for NEC · Minimally invasive surgery for NEC Necrotising Enterocolitis surgical team

8.1 Introduction: When to Operate?

Despite all the uncertainties surrounding exact definitions of NEC and pathophysiology, for the most part, initial clinical management is straightforward. Babies with who meet the criteria for Bell stage I or above receive broad-spectrum IV antibiotics, gastric decompression by means of oro-gastric or nasogastric tube and nil enteral nutrition for a number of days. Arguably, the most difficult question in the management of NEC is *when to perform surgery?* Following on from this, inevitably follows subsequent questions about which surgical procedures to perform. This chapter will consider these questions in turn and then offer two case studies to illustrate the key points.

8.1.1 Should We Operate Sooner?

NEC is managed medically in the first instance. Some infants with NEC deteriorate very rapidly and demonstrate intestinal perforation, meaning that they get surgery relatively early in their disease course. The more common clinical course is that a baby will be managed with medical therapy for 24–48 h and then undergo surgery if indicated. There is some evidence that babies who are operated on earlier have better outcomes [1].

The outcomes of NEC are discussed in detail in Chap. 9 but neurodevelopmental disability is a common sequelae for infants with NEC [2]. The exact mechanism by which NEC leads to neurodevelopmental disability is not known but is probably related to systemic sepsis [3]. The unanswered question here is whether operating earlier would result in better outcomes. Earlier operating would theoretically, at least, mean that the developing brain is exposed to the systemic inflammatory response for a shorter period of time which should result is less brain injury. If this is the case then there is a good argument that operating earlier, but the evidence base for this is currently very limited. Conversely, operating earlier could mean there is a risk of a 'negative laparotomy'—not finding any disease or any intestine that needs resection—which itself could have a detrimental effect in the sense that the infant has been exposed to an unnecessary operation.

For this reason there is a lot of interest in developing clearer criteria for when to operate on NEC that would support clinical decision making.

8.1.2 Absolute Indications

In essence there is one absolute indication for surgery in NEC and that is the presence of pneumoperitoneum, indicating hollow-visceral perforation. In this situation, full thickness necrosis is present at some point in the intestine. These babies do not recover without surgical intervention. Figure 8.1 is a classical x-ray of an infant with perforation secondary to NEC. It should be noted that some infants with a perforation will not have clear evidence of a pneumoperitoneum on a plain anterior-posterior (AP) radiograph. Estimates vary widely on the sensitivity of a plain AP X-ray but potentially 25–50% of infants with a perforation will not have a diagnostic X-ray [4]. Most infants with this kind of radiological appearance will have significant systemic upset and many will already be on inotropic and respiratory support. Where perforation is suspected but not demonstrated, a lateral x-ray (equivalent to an erect chest x-ray in an adult) is most often useful as free intra-peritoneal air is more easily seen. Two different techniques are commonly used for a lateral x-ray in an infant; a lateral-decubitus film or a lateral 'shoot-through' (Fig. 8.2). The images give a slightly different view but provide the same information. In both cases free air may be observed more clearly, in contrast to the liver. This is why a *left* lateral decubitus image is used. There is one pragmatic advantage to the lateral shoot-through x-ray in practice in that the infant does not need to be moved. The x-ray machine is simply re-orientated. For a lateral decubitus image, the patient needs to be rolled on to their side and left in position for 15–20 min in order to obtain the optimal image. In most babies this is not an issue but can be difficult in the most unwell babies who do not tolerate being moved very well.

Fig. 8.1 Abdominal
Radiograph showing
Necrotising enterocolitis
with perforation. Extensive
pneumotosis intestinalis is
visible on the right side.
Rigler's sign is
demonstrated on the left
indicating the presence of a
pneumoperitoneum. The
pneumoperitoneum is
confirmed by the free gas
evident overlying the liver
(Supine film)

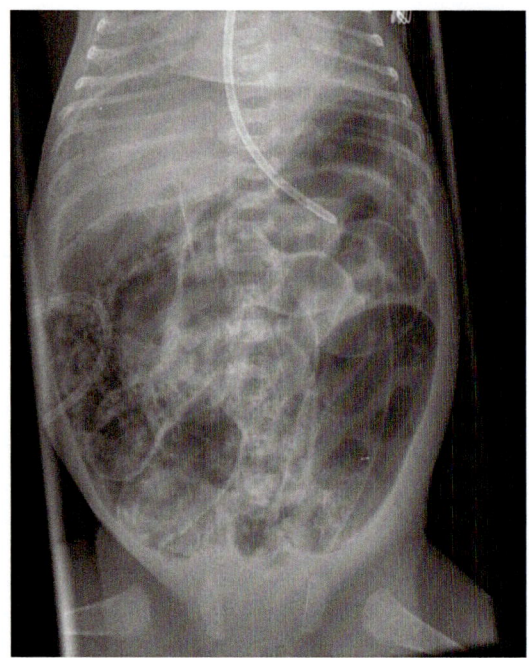

Fig. 8.2 Two approaches
to obtaining a lateral
abdominal radiograph: (**a**)
Shows the left lateral
decubitus position. The
image can be taken both
AP and PA. (**b**) Shows a
lateral shoot-through. The
patient remains in the
supine position but the
x-ray emitter and receiver
are placed to the sides

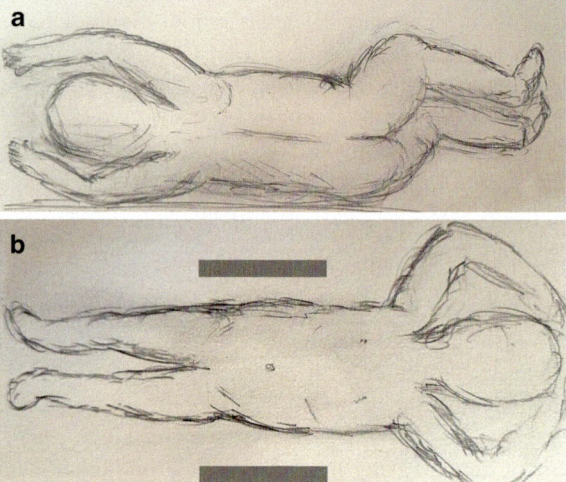

It could be argued that there is a second absolute indication for surgery and that
is the presence of a palpable abdominal mass. Many of these babies have a 'contained perforation' and then develop an inflammatory mass. The phrase 'contained
perforation' describes a full thickness injury to the intestine but with minimal contamination of intestinal contents as the spillage is 'contained' by an inflammatory
response. Again, this is a condition that requires surgical correction. Typically these
babies have a more insidious course and often are less unwell systemically.

8.1.3 Relative Indications

In terms of the decision to operate, the presence of free air is very straightforward; whilst it is not always clear which procedure should be performed the need for intervention is clear-cut. In the absence of a pneumoperitoneum, the decision to operate is more complex.

The phrase that is often used is *failed medical management*. This lacks a clear definition. Many clinicians would consider surgery in an infant who has not improved after 48–72 h of treatment. A deteriorating infant is also one who may well need surgery. In practice, regular clinical assessment is critical.

8.1.3.1 The 'Fixed-Loop' Sign

In health, the intestine is always active. Peristalsis enables gas and liquid contents of the intestine to progress through and the exact position of any given small bowel loop is quite variable. This means that the intestinal gas pattern should not be the same on abdominal x-rays taken at different times.

The 'fixed-loop' sign refers to an area of small bowel that has the same appearance on sequential x-rays. The implication of such a loop is that there is a specific area of small bowel that is not undergoing normal peristalsis. Several papers have reported that the presence of a fixed-loop is a sign of impending perforation and thus an indication for surgery.

A fixed bowel loop is defined as *A dilated intestinal segment with the same location and configuration on serial abdominal x-rays taken at least 24 h apart* [5]. It has been shown that the presence of a fixed bowel loop is strongly associated with increased mortality and the need for surgery [5].

8.1.4 Other Means of Identifying 'Surgical Disease'

A recent systematic review looked back at all of the NEC literature to date that examined this question. It found more than 35 systems for identifying surgical disease, including scoring systems based on multiple factors, radiological markers (in addition to those already discussed) and single biomarkers [6]. The following sections describe the current evidence. There is data to support the use of some or all of these to evaluate babies with NEC. However, currently there is not a biomarker that can be used as a definitive measure for either diagnosing NEC or deciding which babies need surgical intervention. Some of these tests are routinely performed and therefore can support the clinical decision-making. Others are not part of practice at present, and in general, would need better evidence of effectiveness in order to be adopted into routine clinical practice.

8.1.4.1 Platelet Count

Thrombocytopenia is a classical feature of NEC [7]. There is some evidence that both a rapid drop in platelets (i.e. a drop of greater than 150×10^9/L in 24 h reaching a level of 100×10^9/L or less) and severe thrombocytopenia are positive predictors of the need for surgical intervention.

8.1.4.2 C-Reactive Protein

The opsonin, C-reactive protein (CRP) is routinely used as a non-specific inflammatory marker in many areas of practice. In neonates, even small rises in CRP can be an important indicator of developing sepsis. In the context of NEC, higher levels of CRP do correlate with more severe disease and can aid the decision to perform surgery. However, to date, there is insufficient evidence of how precisely this could be done. When, in the disease process, CRP should be measured and what levels should prompt intervention are both unclear. In the absence of such data, CRP is part of the clinical assessment but not currently a practically useful biomarker on its own.

8.1.4.3 Intestinal Fatty-Acid-Binding Protein

Intestinal fatty acid–binding protein (i-FABP) is ubiquitously expressed in the small intestine. Its role includes transporting lipids from the intestinal lumen into enterocytes. When intestinal injury occurs, i-FABP is released into the circulation and serum levels increase. It is subsequently excreted in the urine. Hence, there has been a lot of interest in the potential of i-FABP in NEC.

There is good evidence that levels of i-FABP correlate with the extent of intestinal injury. Different studies have proposed different thresholds but theoretically, it would be possible to use i-FABP as an indicator for surgery. However, it is not currently an option in clinical practice as the test is not routinely available and takes several hours to run. By the time the result of the i-FABP test is available, it is often no longer relevant.

8.1.4.4 Interleukin-6

Interleukin-6 (IL-6) is often considered alongside pro-inflammatory cytokines like TNF-α and IL-1 as they are seen to rise together in response to insult. IL-6 itself has both pro-inflammatory and anti-inflammatory effects. Increased levels of IL-6 are seen in NEC at the tissue level [8] and in the serum in response to sepsis [9]. This biological role implies a potential for clinical use as a biomarker. There are a small number of studies that suggest it might be useful in this context but the data are limited and it is not routine practice.

8.1.4.5 Serum Amyloid A

Serum amyloid A (SAA) is an acute phase protein, which rises within hours of an inflammatory stimulus. It has a very different function to CRP but in terms of a marker of inflammation can be thought of in much the same way. The data is very limited but SAA may be usable as an indicator of the need for surgery but its effectiveness thus far has proven to be limited.

8.1.4.6 Procalcitocin

Procalcitocin is a precursor of the hormone calcitonin. It also appears to have an entirely different function in the context of inflammation and it has been shown that it rises, specifically in response to bacterial infection [10]. An inflammatory marker that is specific for bacterial infection has a lot of theoretical applications, including in the context of NEC. There is some data to suggest that procalcitonin could be an effective biomarker of the need for surgical intervention but it is not currently widely used.

8.1.4.7 Lactate

Serum lactate (usually measured via blood gas analysis) is a routine part of clinical assessment. The molecular biology is well understood as the switch from aerobic respiration to anaerobic within the cells produces lactic acid. As such, it rises in a huge range of physiological and pathological situations and indeed a significant rise is often a very useful indicator of disease severity in the acute setting. However, published data from retrospective studies shows that lactate on its own is not effective as a biomarker of the need for surgery.

8.1.5 Metabolic Derangement 7 Score

As described above, single biomarkers or clinical findings are often not discriminatory between babies with NEC who will recover with medical and supportative therapy only and those that require surgery. As a consequence, scoring systems that combine multiple factors have been proposed for identifying the need for surgery. The Metabolic derangement (MD-7) score is one such system [11].

MD-7 consists—as the name implies—of seven criteria, each scoring one point. A score of three of more is considered an indication for surgery. It is designed to be used in babies without pneumoperitoneum and therefore without a clear-cut reason to operate. The sensitivity of MD-7 is reported as 92% with a specificity of 83.1% [6].

The seven criteria are: *positive blood culture, acidosis, bandemia, thrombocytopenia, hyponatremia, hypotension, and neutropenia.* (Bandemia is a condition in which the neutrophilc count consists of 10% band cells. Band cells are a type of immature neutrophil). These are each used as a binary measure—if present they score one point and zero if absent.

The Score for Neonatal Acute Physiology Perinatal Extension-II (SNAPPE-II) has also been proposed in this context. A direct comparison showed it was not as effective as MD-7 [12].

In general, such scoring systems are not routinely used in clinical practice but there is scope for them to aid clinical decision-making here, especially as institutional studies have shown improved outcomes in units that used the MD-7 [13].

8.1.6   Imaging Methods to Identify Surgical Disease: The Role of Ultrasound?

The plain abdominal radiograph remains the standard investigation in NEC. In addition to this, multiple radiological modalities have been suggested as potentially useful in the management of NEC. Radionucleotide scans, computer topography (CT) and magnetic resonance imaging (MRI) have all been reported as potentially useful but it is abdominal ultrasound that shows the most promise in this area.

Increasing evidence supports the use of abdominal ultrasound scanning (USS) in order to identify which patients with NEC require surgery. The main limitation of USS is that it is an operator-dependent technique and the level of experience of the sonographer clearly effects the ability to obtain diagnostic images. Despite this, many studies have shown that USS can identify surgical disease where clinical uncertainty exists.

There are a number of features of NEC that can be visualised on USS which can be used as relative or absolute indicators for surgery. These include pneumotosis, portal venous gas, pneumoperitoneum, intestinal dilatation, intestinal wall thickening, the presence of ascites and complex fluid collections. Some of these features are commonly found on plain x-ray but may be evident with USS when not visible on a plain film. USS can also identify focal absent peristalsis and absent bowel wall perfusion. These latter two signs are very highly associated with the need for surgical intervention and may be the most useful, as they are features only seen on USS and not visualised on X-ray.

The use of USS has not been widely adopted. This probably reflects the inevitable learning curve as sonographers need to gain enough experience to make clinical decision-making possible. This should improve over time. USS is widely available, cheap and non-invasive. There is a good case for performing a bed-side USS on all babies with suspected NEC, certainly in any baby who is not improving but does not have a clear indication for surgery.

8.1.7   Laparosocopy

Laparoscopy is, of course, a surgical intervention. It involves an anaesthetic and a physiological insult to the patient as well as the practical considerations of clinical teams and equipment needed to perform such a procedure. However, in recent years there has been some interest in the role of laparoscopy as a diagnostic procedure, leading to laparotomy (or drain insertion) if indicated.

Various single centre studies have been published around the use of laparoscopy to inspect the bowel and decide if laparotomy is indicated. These include gasless laparoscopic techniques. Unsurprisingly, they report up to 100% effectiveness at deciding which infants need intervention. The ability to visualise the bowel makes this very appealing. However, as the authors acknowledge this is very invasive and would not be tolerated in very unstable infants [14]. It remains to be seen whether this becomes more widely adopted as part of the surgical assessment and management of infants with NEC.

8.1.8   When Should We Intervene Surgically?

The absolute indication for surgery is clear. Relative indications for surgery remain challenging. If outcomes were the same, regardless of the timing of surgery then it would be a straight-forward matter of monitoring a patient and operating only when it became clear that surgery was needed.

The evidence in this area is very limited but Bethell et al. (2021) reported that outcomes were notably worse in babies who underwent surgery later as they had 'failed medical management' compared to infants who presented with a pneumoperitoneum and had prompt surgery [1]. In this relatively small dataset, there was a much higher mortality in babies in the 'failed medical management' group. Conversely, a systematic review on the timing of surgery and outcomes shows there is almost no evidence in this area [15]. In the context of trauma, there is strong evidence that intervening early to arrest the effects of inflammation and physiological upset is critical to ensuring a good outcome [16] so undoubtedly this is a question that needs answering.

The counter argument to operating earlier is that there is the possibility of finding no clear demarcation within the intestine and therefore no clear benefit from performing a laparotomy. This means exposing a baby to the physiological upset and risks of surgery without a clear benefit. There is also a logistical challenge in that many infants who develop NEC are in neonatal units without surgeons on site and will therefore need to be transferred in order to be assessed by a surgeon.

Chapter 10 is dedicated to the future of NEC and focuses on novel treatment options. Research in this area is critically important but clinical research on current practice and potential ways to improve outcomes are also important. Ways to identify which infants need surgery earlier could lead to better outcomes, both in terms of mortality but also neurodevelopmental disability. Similarly, in the absence of clearer indications, should the threshold for surgery be lower? Should more babies undergo laparotomy, accepting the risk of a 'negative' laparotomy? There is very limited data on this at present but there is a lot of evidence that suggests timing of surgery is important and therefore this warrants careful study and potentially a change in practice.

8.2 Anaesthetic Considerations

Anaesthesia in premature infants is complex and requires specialist skills. The immature cardiovascular system and the predisposition of the respiratory system to brochio-pulmonary dysplasia and apnoea create specific challenges [17].

Where-ever possible, infants requiring surgery for NEC should be pre-optimised. This is often not possible as critically ill infants need surgery alongside on-going resuscitation [18]. These babies often require large volumes of IV fluid replacement in addition to maintenance fluids for normoglycaemia.

Many of these babies will need inotropic support prior to an operation. Similarly, it is common to need to introduce them during surgery. Blood loss needs replacement with whole blood (i.e. packed red blood cells, plasma and platelets). This reflects that even if blood loss is relatively small, the overall physiological compromise makes coagulopathy a particular problem.

In addition to standard routine monitoring, central venous pressure and invasive arterial pressure monitoring can be very helpful. Whether they are used or not is most often determined by weighing the benefit of such monitoring against the time needed to secure the central venous and arterial access in a very small infant: it may be inappropriate to delay treatment in order to obtain invasive monitoring. However, body temperature monitoring and active warming measures are essential [18]. It has been shown that preterm babies undergoing surgery have an increased neuroendocrine response and a prolonged surgical stress response (compared to term babies and adults) [19]. For this reason, high dose opioid use at induction may be beneficial to reduce post-operative catabolism caused by the stress response.

Evidence from animal studies suggests that many anaesthetic agents may be toxic to the developing brain and this is an area of on-going research. So far, studies into cognitive abilities have shown no measurable effect of a single anaesthetic in infants [17]. This is an important area of research but it is essentially a moot point as the majority of critically ill infants with NEC will die without operative treatment.

8.3   Laparotomy or Not? The Role of Peritoneal Drains

Peritoneal drainage (PD), as an alternative to laparotomy for NEC with perforation, was first reported by Ein et al. in 1977 [20]. A Penrose drain (named for the American gynaecologist who first described its use) is a soft, flexible tube designed to allow passive drainage. In many of the smallest neonates, the finger from a surgical glove makes an ideal device for this purpose. The aim of a PD is to decompress the abdomen and remove peritoneal toxic effluents without the need for open surgery. PD has become an established alternative to a laparotomy in haemodynamically unstable infants who will not tolerate open surgery (or potentially transport to another centre for surgery). It is also a less aggressive and sometimes definitive first line treatment [21].

In practical terms, a small incision, insertion of a soft tube and placement of a retaining skin suture is the work of only a couple of minutes and is well tolerated by unstable infants. Exact position in the abdomen is unimportant but many surgeons will choose the left iliac fossa (opposite McBurney's point) as a suitable site. Placing a drain on the left minimises the risk of liver injury. A PD can also be placed under local anaesthesia, avoiding the need for heavy sedation or a general anaesthetic.

Several studies have looked at the specific question of how PD compares to laparotomy. Most of these are observational studies but there have been three randomised-control trials (RCT) as well. It should be noted that many of these studies include patients with SIP as well as NEC. From a surgical perspective, the acute management is much the same but they are different disease processes and therefore outcomes are not necessarily comparable.

A recent systematic review showed that combining the three published RCTs showed no difference in survival between babies who had PD compared to those who had laparotomy as their primary intervention [21]. Pooled data from the observational studies did suggest lower survival among babies who had PD. There is of course a higher risk of bias in these studies. In order to answer this question definitively, power calculations suggest that a much larger RCT would be needed which is probably not practical.

It is therefore a viable option to place a PD drain in babies with evidence of perforation. At least 50% of such babies are likely to need a laparotomy subsequently [22] which is why it is often viewed as a temporising measure rather than definitive treatment. However, such data does suggest that some babies who have a PD will not need a laparotomy as PD can be definitive treatment.

Opinions on the role of PD in perforated NEC vary. It certainly has its place—especially in very unstable infants who are not good candidates for a laparotomy. Similarly it may be a very good option in babies who would need transfer prior to a laparotomy and are not likely to tolerate being moved. Placement of a PD certainly does not commit an infant to needing a laparotomy but the data also shows that in a majority, it is not definitive either and surgery will be needed in the following days.

8.4   Principles of Surgery in NEC

The principles of NEC surgery involve bowel inspection, resection of necrotic bowel, peritoneal lavage and restoration of bowel continuity or stoma formation. In the most unwell patients, minimising operative time should also be a priority.

Physiologically, these infants are compromised by a combination of factors. Necrotic bowel drives systemic upset and an acute systemic inflammatory response. Often abdominal distension due to bowel dilatation and fluid accumulation also causes respiratory compromise. As such, the priorities with a laparotomy are to relieve the respiratory embarrassment by draining fluid and gas from the abdominal cavity and then remove the necrotic intestine that is driving the systemic upset and secondary organ compromise.

NEC surgery is very variable. Some infants will have a mass and contained perforation. These infants are usually not as systemically unwell. Many infants have NEC and perforation in one specific area of the intestine, whilst others will have multiple areas of NEC, potentially in both the large and small intestine. This is why inspection of all of the small bowel is important. Conversely, inspection of the colon is not always desirable as this may require extensive mobilisation which can cause significant bleeding. It may be better to defunction the colon (by performing an ileostomy) without attempting a colectomy in the first instance.

From a technical perspective, surgery on preterm babies is different to surgery in term neonates. The small size of the infants is an obvious consideration. In addition, the intestine and mesentery is more fragile and does not tolerate handling as well, necessitating extra care from the operating surgeon. Moreover, the preterm liver is particularly susceptible to haemorrhage. This is crucial as control of a sub-capsular liver bleed can be very difficult and the low circulating blood volume of these neonates means that their tolerance of blood loss is correspondingly low.

8.5   Stoma Versus Primary Anastomosis

Necrotic small bowel needs to be resected. Once this has been done there is a decision to be made about the bowel continuity. It could be considered a classical approach to perform a stoma and mucus fistula with an aim to restore intestinal continuity at a later stage as primary anastomosis was once considered a hazardous option due to the risk of anastomotic leak [23]. This remains an important option in NEC and may well be the best option in some babies. It has the advantage of avoiding the risk of anastomotic complications in an unstable patient and can shorten operative time. However, there are consequences of performing a stoma that should be properly weighed against these advantages.

One study showed that over 80% of infants with a stoma will suffer at least one complication prior to the stoma being closed [24]. Stomas complications include stenosis, parastoma hernia and prolapse as well as skin excoriation from contact with effluent. Many of these will require surgery—potentially refashioning of the stoma, if they are not ready reversal.

Management of nutrition and fluid balance is also often more complicated in babies with a stoma. Babies with a stoma show slower rates of growth [25] and increased need for parenteral nutrition (PN). Indeed, perhaps a fifth of babies with a stoma require PN until the stoma is closed [24].

The location of the stoma has a bearing on the likely difficulties: a distal ileostomy is preferable to a proximal jejunostomy. With a distal ileostomy, the entire (residual) small intestine remains in continuity and hence the infant has the full absorptive capacity of the small bowel. The (effective) absence of the colon does have an effect on fluid balance and nutrition but undoubtedly the small intestine is much more important for enteral function. Many of these babies manage well with a stoma. Conversely a 'high' stoma, formed in the proximal small bowel inevitably means that the fluids losses are higher and the absorption of nutrients is correspondingly lower.

Several published studies support primary anastomosis as a safe option in neonates with NEC requiring bowel resection, including VLBW infants [26, 27]. Whilst clearly not applicable to all situations, the fact that primary anastomosis is shown to be safe and effective in general in NEC is important. Infants with a stoma will have sequelae that may be significant and hence avoiding a stoma is definitely desirable, if it is possible.

If a baby does have a stoma, the ideal timing for closure is also unclear. A survey of practice in the UK showed that most surgeons favoured an 'early' closure around 6 weeks of age. It also showed that the weight of the infant was the most commonly used factor for deciding when to perform stoma closure. This is an important point; infants who are failing to thrive due to the stoma often show significant improvement once the stoma is closed [28].

Stoma formation is definitely an important option in NEC surgery but their use is not without its implications. There is a good body of evidence to show that performing a primary anastomosis is a safe and reasonable option in many situations and avoids the not insignificant problems that a stoma can cause.

8.6 Laparostomy, 'Clip and Crop,' and the 'Damage Control Approach'

'Laparostomy' is the term for an operation where the peritoneal cavity is opened anteriorly and deliberately left open. The term 'open abdomen' is often used to describe such patients. The abdominal contents are exposed and therefore are protected with a temporary covering.

Laparostomies are used in severely ill or injured patients to fascilitate healing and prevent complications—such as abdominal compartment syndrome [29]. In the early part of the twenty-first century, the use of laparostomy has become routine in severe trauma. The emphasis here is less on the risk of abdominal compartment syndrome and more on minimising the physiological insult [16, 30]. Patients who suffer major trauma can easily develop a deadly triad of acidosis, hypothermia and coagulopathy leading to multi-organ failure. Extensive surgery, as historically performed, whilst able to restore anatomy, only worsened the physiological situation which meant these patients still suffered a high mortality, despite the best efforts of the medical teams.

The use of laparostomy in NEC surgery was first reported in the 1990s [31] but, among other things, the evidence from trauma surgery has led to a renewed interest in this approach to severely unwell infants with NEC. Vaughan et al. described their 'clip and drop' technique whereby they managed three babies with NEC (and two with malrotation and volvulus) with a laparostomy [31]. Each patient had extensive necrosis, requiring multiple resections. They performed delayed primary anastomoses 48 to 72 h later.

The extensive use of a so-called 'damage control approach' in trauma has led to renewed interest in its utility is other contexts, including very unwell neonates with intestinal perforation. It is a first glance, little different from previous reports but strictly speaking the concept of *damage control* is more than just the use of a laparostomy. It is a focus on restoring physiology as quickly as possible with the surgical procedure being part of the resuscitation process. Correction of anatomical disruption is not a consideration in the acute setting. The focus is on removing necrotic bowel, peritoneal lavage at the same time as maintaining and correcting physiological upset with active warming and the administration of blood products and fluids as needed.

A modification on the dressing used by the British military in major trauma, termed a 'mini-Bastion sandwich' is a simple technique that works well in small babies [30]. An inner layer of perforated plastic is placed over the bowel to protect it. Gauze is then layed on top of this. A suction tube is placed next with a second layer of gauze over the top. The 'sandwich' dressing is then completed with an airtight dressing over the top. The tube is then connected to low pressure suction. This arrangement is important for maintaining sterility—the removal of fluid from the dressing ensures that the air tight layer remains dry and does not start to lift-off [30].

The primary purpose of a damage-control approach is to minimise the physiological insult in the first instance with definitive surgery being performed at a later point when the patient's overall condition has improved and inotropes are no longer needed. The secondary benefit is the ability to inspect the bowel a second time allowing clearer demarcation of disease in the bowel and thus potentially a more conservative resection than might otherwise be possible. This also allows primary anastomosis to be considered in all infants, even if multiple resections are required.

Whilst this approach is—as Vaughan et al. [31] put it—an important part of the armament of a neonatal surgeon, there is not currently sufficient data to show superior outcomes for these neonates. The use of laparostomy is not without negative consequences, especially if closure is delayed beyond 72 h [29]. There is also a pragmatic consideration that some of the a babies who have a laparostomy will die without undergoing a second-look procedure and thus a strategy for how to manage these infants is necessary.

8.7   Case Studies

8.7.1   Case Study 1

This case involves a 18 day old male infant who was a twin and born at 29 weeks completed gestation. His birth weight was 1020 g. He was born by emergency cae-sarean section and no antenatal steroids were given. He was intubated and ventilated on day 1 but was extubated 3 days later. He was fully fed with a mixture of maternal breast milk and formula. His current weight is 1100 g. On day 17 of life he deterio-rated, with abdominal distension and bilious aspirates. His abdominal x-ray showed non-specific findings with some gas filled loops but no diagnostic features. He had the following blood results:

Full blood count		
Haemoglobin	102 g/L	(134–199)
Haematocrit	0.61 L/L	(0.32–0.65)
White cell count	14.0×10^9/L	(6.0–21.0)
Platelets	124×10^9/L	(150–450)
Differential White cell count		
Neutrophils	11.0×10^9/L	(1.5–5.4)
Lymphocytes	2.4×10^9/L	(2.8–9.1)
Monocytes	0.3×10^9/L	(0.1–1.7)
Biochemistry		
Creatinine	22 mmol/L	(16–47)
Urea	8.0 mmol/L	(1.1–8.0)
Sodium	136 mmol/L	(136–146)
Potassium	4.1 mmol/L	(3.5–5.3)
C-reactive protein	17 mg/L	(<5.0)
References ranges vary by laboratory		

Enteral feeds were stopped and the NG tube placed on free drainage. IV antibiot-ics were started. Supplementary oxygen was given via nasal prongs at 1 L/min. Twenty four hours later, he had deteriorated to the point of needing invasive ventila-tion. His abdomen is more distended and he does not tolerate handling. When exam-ined, his heart rate falls to around 80 beats/min before recovering. Over the past few hours he has required increasing ventilator pressures to maintain oxygen saturations and clearance of CO_2. He currently has a PEEP of 7 cm H_2O and a volume-control mode of ventilation is delivering a peak pressure of 25 cm H_2O.

Q1. How should he be managed at this stage?

A1. *The clinical picture has changed and there has been a deterioration in this infant's condition at this point. His blood tests and abdominal x-ray should be repeated. Given that he has increased distension, signs of abdominal tenderness* *(poor tolerance of examination) and systemic deterioration, intestinal perforation should be considered. If a standard AP x-ray is equivocal, a lateral x-ray will be needed. If his respiratory function deteriorates further then HFOV should be considered, this will be guided by the blood gas results. He may need inotropic support.*

His blood results and AP abdominal film are shown below:

Full blood count		
Haemoglobin	98 g/L	(134–199)
Haematocrit	0.63 L/L	(0.32–0.65)
White Cell Count	23.0×10^9/L	(6.0–21.0)
Platelets	56×10^9/L	(150–450)
Differential White cell count		
Neutrophils	15.0×10^9/L	(1.5–5.4)
Lymphocytes	2.2×10^9/L	(2.8–9.1)
Monocytes	0.3×10^9/L	(0.1–1.7)
Biochemistry		
Creatinine	35 mmol/L	(16–47)
Urea	8.8 mmol/L	(1.1–8.0)
Sodium	131 mmol/L	(136–146)
Potassium	4.5 mmol/L	(3.5–5.3)
C-reactive protein	101 mg/L	(<5.0)
References ranges vary by laboratory		

See Fig. 8.3.

Q2. What does this abdominal x-ray show? How should this be interpreted in the context of the infant's overall clinical status and blood results?

A2: This Anterio-posterior abdominal film shows an NG-tube in the stomach, a right saphenous long-line with the tip in a central position and patchy-changes in the bases of both lungs. The abdomen is relatively gas-less, consistent with significant ascites and fluid-filled gas loops. There is a lucency centrally in the upper abdomen.

The overall picture is one of an infant whose disease has progressed, even though there are no absolute diagnostic features of NEC on this x-ray. The rapid rise in CRP and fall in platelets is consistent with NEC and suggestive that surgery may be needed. A lateral radiograph is indicated.

The lateral abdominal x-ray is shown below (Fig. 8.4).

Q3. What are the next steps in the management of this baby?

A3: This lateral-decubitus film shows free gas within the abdomen demonstrating that there is an intestinal perforation. This child will need surgical intervention. In most cases, a laparotomy may be performed but placement of a peritoneal drain is a reasonable alternative. This infants is anaemic and has thrombocytopenia and therefore will need blood products prior to surgical intervention. If the infant is not in a surgical centre then safe transfer will need to be arranged.

Fig. 8.3 Case study
1—abdominal x-ray

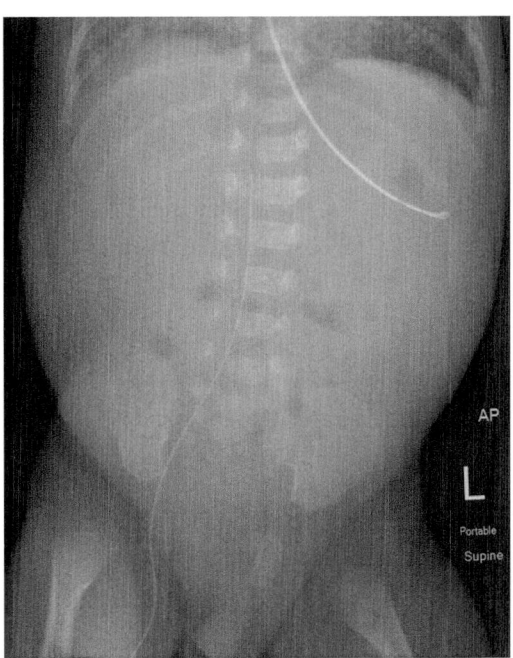

Fig. 8.4 Case study 1—
lateral decubitas abdominal
x-ray

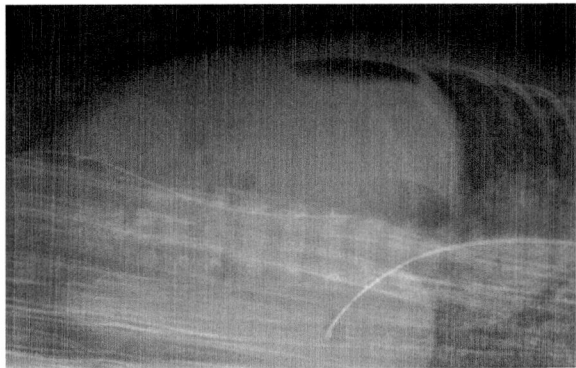

8.7.2   Case Study 2

An infant born at 24 weeks and 2 days gestation developed clear signs of NEC on day 11 of life. Enteral feeding was stopped, his NG tube was placed on free drainage and broad spectrum antibiotics were started. He required intubation and ventilation at this stage. The following day, he had deteriorated further and inotropic support with both dobutamine and dopamine was started. Abdominal radiography did not show clear evidence of perforation and an abdominal ultrasound was not available. The decision was made to proceed to laparotomy given the clear diagnosis of NEC

Fig. 8.5 Case study 2—
intraoperative findings

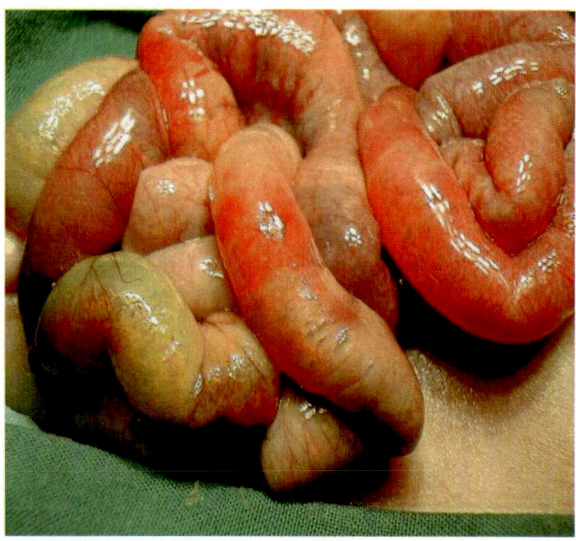

and rapid clinical deterioration. He was 930 g at time of surgery. The figure below
shows the operative findings (Fig. 8.5).

Q1. What does this image show?

*A1: This image shows all of the small bowel has been eviscerated for inspection.
No site of perforation is evident in this image. The image shows an area of ischaemic necrosis with impending perforation as well as some healthy small bowel and
some areas of disease which may recover.*

Q2. What are the options for surgical management at this point?

*A2: The whole small bowel needs to be carefully inspected. The area of necrosis
needs to be resected. There may be other areas that also require resection. Given
that the infant is currently on inotropes, primary anastomosis is hazardous.
Formation of a stoma is an option. Damage control surgery should also be considered. Removal of frankly necrotic bowel, followed by washout of the abdomen and
formation of a laparostomy has two advantages in this situation. Firstly, it can be
completed in 20–30 min and therefore minimises the operative time in a baby with
significant physiological compromise. Secondly, the areas of bowel that may recover
can be left and reviewed at the second operation. This minimises the need for resection and may allow a delayed primary anastomosis.*

References

1. Bethell G, Knight M, Hall N. Surgical necrotizing enterocolitis: association between surgical indication, timing, and outcomes. J Pediatr Surg. 2021;56(10):1785–90. https://doi.
   org/10.1016/j.jpedsurg.2021.04.028.
2. Jones IH, Hall NJ. Contemporary outcomes for infants with necrotizing enterocolitis—a systematic review. J Pediatr. 2020;220:86–92. https://doi.org/10.1016/j.jpeds.2019.11.011.

3. Lu J, Martin C, Claud E. Neurodevelopmental outcome of infants who develop necrotizing enterocolitis: the gut-brain axis. Semin Perinatol. 2023;47(1):151694. https://doi.
   org/10.1016/j.semperi.2022.151694.
4. Devos AS, Baert AL, Blickman JG. Radiological imaging of the digestive tract in infants and
   children. Heidelberg: Springer Berlin; 2007.
5. Muller A, Schurink M, Bos A, Hulzebos C, Martijn A, Hulscher J, Kooi E. Clinical importance of a fixed bowel loop in the treatment of necrotizing enterocolitis. Neonatology.
   2014;105(1):33–8. https://doi.org/10.1159/000355064.
6. Bethell GJ, Jones IH, Battersby C, Knight M, Hall NJ. Methods of identifying surgical necrotizing enterocolitis—a systematic review and meta-analysis. J Pediatr. 2024; https://doi.
   org/10.1038/s41390-024-03292-3.
7. Ragazzi S, Pierro A, Peters M, Fasoli L, Eaton S. Early full blood count and severity of disease in neonates with necrotizing enterocolitis. Pediatr Surg Int. 2003;19(5):376–9. https://doi.
   org/10.1007/s00383-003-1014-5.
8. Cho SX, Berger PJ, Nold-Petry CA, Nold MF. The immunological landscape in necrotising
   enterocolitis. Expert Rev Mol Med. 2016;18:e12. https://doi.org/10.1017/erm.2016.13.
9. Kim YH, Yoon DW, Kim JH, Lee JH, Lim CH. Effect of remote ischemic post-conditioning
   on systemic inflammatory response and survival rate in lipopolysaccharide-induced systemic
   inflammation model. J Inflamm. 2014;11:16. https://doi.org/10.1186/1476-9255-11-16.
10. Samsudin I, Vasikaran S. Clinical utility and measurement of procalcitonin. Clin Biochem
    Rev. 2017;38(2):59–68.
11. Tepas JJ 3rd, Sharma R, Leaphart CL, Celso BG, Pieper P, Esquivia-Lee V. Timing of sur-
    gical intervention in necrotizing enterocolitis can be determined by trajectory of metabolic
    derangement. J Pediatr Surg. 2010;45(2):310–3.; ; discussion 3–4. https://doi.org/10.1016/j.
    jpedsurg.2009.10.069.
12. Fijas M, Vega M, Xie X, Kim M, Havranek T. SNAPPE-II and MDAS scores as predictors for
    surgical intervention in very low birth weight neonates with necrotizing enterocolitis. J Matern
    Fetal Neonatal Med. 2023;36(1):2148096. https://doi.org/10.1080/14767058.2022.2148096.
13. Tepas J, Leaphart C, Plumley D, Sharma R, Celso B, Pieper P, et al. Trajectory of meta-
    bolic derangement in infants with necrotizing enterocolitis should drive timing and technique
    of surgical intervention. J Am Coll Surg. 2010;210(5):847–52. https://doi.org/10.1016/j.
    jamcollsurg.2010.01.008.
14. Numanoglu A, Millar A. Necrotizing enterocolitis: early conventional and fluorescein lapa-
    roscopic assessment. J Pediatr Surg. 2011;46(2):348–51. https://doi.org/10.1016/j.jpedsurg.
    2010.11.021.
15. Duric B, Gray C, Alexander A, Naik S, Haffenden V, Yardley I. Effect of time of diagnosis to
    surgery on outcome, including long-term neurodevelopmental outcome, in necrotizing entero-
    colitis. Pediatr Surg Int. 2022;39(1):2. https://doi.org/10.1007/s00383-022-05283-z.
16. Bowley D, Barker P, Boffard K. Damage control surgery—concepts and practice. J R Army
    Med Corps. 2000;146(3):176–82. https://doi.org/10.1136/jramc-146-03-05.
17. Subramaniam R. Anaesthetic concerns in preterm and term neonates. Indian J Anaesth.
    2019;63(9):771–9. https://doi.org/10.4103/ija.IJA_591_19.
18. Sodhi P, Fiset P. Necrotizing enterocolitis. Continuing Ed Anaesth Crit Care Pain.
    2024;12(1):1–4. https://doi.org/10.1093/bjaceaccp/mkr043.
19. Anand K, Sippell W, Aynsley-Green A. Randomised trial of fentanyl anaesthesia in preterm
    babies undergoing surgery: effects on the stress response. Lancet. 1987;1(8527):62–6. https://
    doi.org/10.1016/s0140-6736(87)90065-1.
20. Ein S, Marshal DG, Girvan D. Peritoneal drainage under local anesthesia for perfo-
    rations from necrotizing enterocolitis. J Pediatr Surg. 1977;12(6):963–7. https://doi.
    org/10.1016/0022-3468(77)90607-8.
21. Solis-Garcia G, Pierro A, Jasani B. Laparotomy versus peritoneal drainage as primary treat-
    ment for surgical necrotizing enterocolitis or spontaneous intestinal perforation in preterm
    neonates: a systematic review and meta-analysis. Children. 2023;10(7):1170. https://doi.
    org/10.3390/children10071170.

22. Blakely M, Tyson J, Lally K, Hintz S, Eggleston B, Stevenson D, et al. Initial laparotomy versus peritoneal drainage in extremely low birthweight infants with surgical necrotizing enterocolitis or isolated intestinal perforation: a multicenter randomized clinical trial. Ann Surg. 2021;274(4):e370–80. https://doi.org/10.1097/SLA.0000000000005099.
23. Pierro A, Hall N. Surgical treatments of infants with necrotizing enterocolitis. Semin Neonatol. 2003;8(3):223–32. https://doi.org/10.1016/S1084-2756(03)00025-3.
24. Wolf L, Gfroerer S, Fiegel H, Rolle U. Complications of newborn enterostomies. World J Clin Cases. 2018;6(16):1101–10. https://doi.org/10.12998/wjcc.v6.i16.1101.
25. Pan P. The outcome of late versus early ileostomy closure at low body weight. J Indian Assoc Pediatr Surg. 2022;27(2):204–8. https://doi.org/10.4103/jiaps.JIAPS_369_20.
26. Singh M, Owen A, Gull S, Morabito A, Bianchi A. Surgery for intestinal perforation in preterm neonates: anastomosis vs stoma. J Pediatr Surg. 2006;41(4):725–9. https://doi.org/10.1016/j.jpedsurg.2005.12.017.
27. Hall N, Curry J, Drake D, Spitz L, Kiely E, Pierro A. Resection and primary anastomosis is a valid surgical option for infants with necrotizing enterocolitis who weigh less than 1000 g. Arch Surg. 2005;140(12):1149–51. https://doi.org/10.1001/archsurg.140.12.1149.
28. Ducey J, Kennedy A, Linsell L, Woolfall K, Hall N, Gale C, et al. Timing of neonatal stoma closure: a survey of health professional perspectives and current practice. Arch Dis Child Fetal Neonatal Ed. 2022;107(4):448–50. https://doi.org/10.1136/archdischild-2021-322040.
29. Leppäniemi A. Laparostomy: why and when? Crit Care. 2010;14(2):216. https://doi.org/10.1186/cc8857.
30. Arul G, Singh M, Ali A, Gee O. Damage control surgery in neonates: lessons learned from the battlefield. J Pediatr Surg. 2019;54(10):2069–74. https://doi.org/10.1016/j.jpedsurg.2019.04.001.
31. Vaughan W, Grosfeld J, West K, Scherer L, Villamizar E, Rescorla F. Avoidance of stomas and delayed anastomosis for bowel necrosis: the 'clip and drop-back' technique. J Pediatr Surg. 1996;31(4):542–5. https://doi.org/10.1016/s0022-3468(96)90492-3.

Chapter 9
Outcomes of Necrotising Enterocolitis

Contents

Abstract Necrotising enterocolitis remains a great scourge of neonatal intensive care units. Despite decades of research and significant improvements in neonatal care, outcomes following NEC are essentially unchanged.

Overall, approximate one in four neonates who contract NEC (Bell stage IIa or higher) will not survive. The mortality of infants who require surgical intervention for NEC is around 30%, rising to over 50% in the most premature infants with surgical disease.

Survivors often have significant neurodevelopmental disability with widely ranging reported rates. The true prevalence of severe disability following NEC is likely to be around a third. Similarly there is a high incidence of intestinal failure.

A significant minority of infants who have surgery for NEC will still require parenteral nutrition 3 months later and some will need it long-term.

The outcomes of NEC remain poor. Undoubtedly, better treatments for NEC are desperately needed.

Keywords NEC outcomes · Morbidity of NEC · Mortality of NEC · Long-term outcomes of NEC · Neurodevelopmental outcomes in NEC survivors · Growth outcomes in NEC survivors · Gastrointestinal outcomes in NEC survivors Neurological outcomes in NEC survivors · Respiratory outcomes in NEC survivors · Surgical outcomes in NEC survivors · Quality of life in NEC survivors Complications of NEC · NEC-related disabilities · NEC-related neurodevelopmental delay · NEC-related gastrointestinal complications NEC-related respiratory complications · NEC-related surgical complications NEC recurrence rates · Follow-up care for NEC survivors · Prognostic factors in NEC outcomes

9.1   Introduction

Necrotising enterocolitis is an acute illness. An episode of NEC will last a few days. Treatment of the acute episode takes 10 days or so. Some patients will make a complete recovery whilst others have major, life-long sequelae. NEC continues to have a high mortality but it is wrong to solely focus on survival, as a significant proportion of survivors will have long-term effects from their acute episode.

In terms of mortality from NEC, there is a notable late-mortality. A minority of babies who survive to discharge will not survive to 2 years of age. Only measuring in-hospital mortality/survival to discharge therefore does not fully capture NEC mortality.

The long-term outcomes of NEC are of key importance. When considering the effectiveness of any current or future treatment, it is the effect on long-term outcomes that should be assessed. Moreover, for neonatal and surgical teams, counselling parents of affected babies effectively, relies on having appropriate data about what they can realistically expect.

Through an extensive Delphi process with a broad range of stakeholders, a core outcome set for NEC has recently been agreed [1]. The stakeholders included physicians, patients and family representatives. The agreed core outcomes are:

- Mortality
- NEC-related mortality
- Short bowel syndrome
- Quality of life
- Neurodevelopmental impairment

The hope is that going-forward, all studies looking at NEC, especially those involving putative new interventions will report on these outcomes as a way of accurately quantifying the disease burden and allowing comparison between studies.

It is not surprising that mortality tops this list as it remains the case that NEC has a high mortality. The difference between NEC-mortality and all-cause mortality is important as babies afflicted with NEC have a higher mortality from other causes than equivalent neonates who did not contract NEC. In these infants, the causes of death will include chronic lung disease and intestinal failure. Contracting NEC—especially if surgery is required—worsens lung function, increasing the risk of issues in the future. Therefore it is important to consider all-cause mortality when looking at NEC-outcomes.

Quality of life for survivors is, of course, an indispensable outcome measure. How this should be quantified is sadly less straightforward but several validated score-systems exist for adults and children of different ages. Overall though, capturing the other two core outcomes (short-bowel syndrome and neurodevelopmental impairment) will encompass the majority of the life-long morbidity for NEC survivors.

One large study of nearly 10,000 ELBW infants showed a rehospitalisation rate of 35.2% by 18–24 months follow-up. In those infants who had had NEC, the rehospitalisation rate was 46.4% [2]. The reasons for rehospitalisation included respiratory illness, nutritional issues (failure to thrive), seizure disorders and sepsis. In essence, infants who had NEC have the same causes of rehospitalisation as other children born prematurely who did not have NEC. They are simply at a higher risk of needing admission for these reasons.

When considering outcomes for NEC it is important to stratify the affected infants by maturity and severity of disease. Infants with birthweights of less than 750 g have a mortality rate that is three times higher than those weighing between 1250 and 1500 g at birth [3]. Similarly babies requiring surgery for their NEC have more severe disease and would therefore be expected to have worse outcomes.

All of the data described in this chapter corresponds to high-income countries only. Overall neonatal outcomes are dramatically different between high- and low-income countries. In 2019, Europe had an overall neonatal mortality of 5 per 1000 live births compared to 27 per 1000 live births in Sub-Saharan Africa [4]. This difference implies that the incidence of NEC may well be much lower in low-income countries because the population of ELBW and VLBW infants who survive the perinatal period to be at risk of NEC is much smaller. It is also likely that for those who do contract NEC, will also have similarly poorer outcomes. These are rational conclusions but there is a paucity of data for NEC outcomes from low-income countries.

9.2 Intestinal Strictures

NEC is an inflammatory process. Strictures are found throughout the alimentary canal as a secondary phenomenon of inflammation. Gastro-oesophageal reflux can cause oesophagitis and this can lead to oesophageal stricturing. Similarly strictures are a near-universal phenomenon in Crohn's disease. In each case, the detailed pathophysiological mechanism is not fully elucidated. A simplistic model of how strictures form would postulate that scarring results from the inflammatory process. Scars shrink over time. If the scarring is circumferential in a tube, then that tube will narrow. Hence strictures are to be expected in NEC if the affected bowel is not resected.

9.2.1   Incidence of Intestinal Stricture After NEC

Estimates of the incidence show a very wide variation. Work from the 1970s reported published rates varying from 6% to 33% [5]. More recently studies have reported rates of over 50% [6, 7] which is much higher than many would expect from their clinical experience. There may be some differences in definition between studies that accounts for this large variation. For example, whether a radiological or surgical diagnosis of stricture is used. It seems unlikely that this is a full or even major explanation, however. Strictures require treatment with surgery. It is possible that patients have minor strictures that are not operated on but asymptomatic patients do not usually get radiological examination and therefore these strictures would not be detected. So it is less plausible that this difference can be explained by differences in reporting alone. Whatever the exact number, strictures are a common occurrence in babies who have had NEC.

It would be logical to assume that strictures were only seen in babies who's initial episode of NEC was managed conservatively. This is not true, however. Operatively, necrotic intestine is resected and then either a stoma is formed or the bowel is anastomosed. However this does not mean that all of the NEC-affected bowel has been removed. Surgeons will often leave areas of small bowel that are affected if the disease is mild and the intestine is viable. It is not always possible to tell by intra-operative inspection whether any given area of intestine is affected or not. Over the following few days, NEC may continue to develop and these areas can become stenosed in the same way that the intestine narrows in babies with NEC who do not undergo surgery.

9.3   Mortality

There are a large number of studies on the outcomes for NEC. The quoted figures vary enormously. This reflects multiple factors. The case-definition of NEC used varies significantly as well as the definition of mortality. Some studies report survival to discharge, some survival to 2 years. Some report all-cause mortality whilst others only report mortality attributed to NEC. For these reasons—and others—the literature includes very wide estimates of NEC mortality. The data quoted in this section are predominantly from a systematic review

Table 9.1 Overall mortality from NEC

Group		Mortality %
All NEC	All neonates with NEC (Bell 1–3)	15.3
	All neonates with NEC (Bell 2+)	23.5
ELBW and VLBW	Neonates with BW <1500 g (Bell 2+)	30.1
	Neonates with BW <1000 g (Bell 2+)	41.3
Surgical NEC	All neonates with surgical NEC	34.5
	Neonates with BW <1500 g & Surgical NEC	40.5
	Neonates with BW <1000 g & Surgical NEC	50.9

These data are based on meta-analyses of multicentre studies. Each analysis is based on at least 3000 infants (Based on Jones and Hall [8])

published in 2020 which only included large, multicentre series published since 2010 [8].

9.3.1   Overall Mortality

Table 9.1 summarises the mortality. As discussed in previous chapters, a significant number of infants who meet the criteria for Bell stage I, will not actually have NEC. Perhaps even a majority. Therefore it is not surprising that there is a large discrepancy between the mortality in series that include only babies who were Bell stage II or above compared to series that included all babies labelled as NEC. Essentially, including the Bell stage I patients will simply increases the denominator.

Therefore, the overall mortality for confirmed NEC is 23.5% or approximately one in four. Given that the overall survival for premature babies without congenital issues and without NEC is now over 95% this is particularly stark. Even with babies born at 24 weeks, the majority survive.

The survival figures for the most premature babies who contract NEC are correspondingly lower (as would be expected) with around 70% of VLBW infants with NEC surviving and 60% of ELBW infants.

9.3.2   Surgical Mortality

In this context 'surgical disease' or 'surgical NEC' is defined as an infant who received either a laparotomy or an abdominal drain for NEC.

Overall mortality in this group is around 35%, rising to over 40% in VLBW infants and over 50% is the smallest (ELBW) infants.

Having a surgical intervention for NEC is associated with a significantly higher mortality than medically treated NEC.

9.3.3   Late Mortality

Most studies of NEC report in-hospital mortality or 30-day mortality. However, long-term follow-up studies have clearly demonstrated that such data does not fully encompass the mortality associated with contracting NEC. Studies that look at children up to 2 years of age show that many of those that do not survive will be discharged home from their initial episode (or survive beyond 30 days) and then succumb later. This rate of late mortality is between 5% and 30%. Specifically, all-cause mortality measured at 2 years of age in patients diagnosed with NEC is around 6% higher in absolute terms than mortality measured at 30 days (or discharge) [8].

The causes of death will be the same as for other children born prematurely, namely: respiratory, sepsis or complications secondary to intestinal failure. What these data clearly show is that babies that are successfully discharged are not fully 'out-of-the-woods.'

9.3.4   Unanswered Questions

The data described here is the best currently available, being based on large multi-centre cohorts. It provides the detailed information to allow counselling of families when an NEC diagnosis is made and is an aid to decision-making. However it is certainly not complete and there are some key questions that remain unanswered.

A mortality of around a third for all babies requiring surgery needs to be understood in context. It does not immediately suggest that the surgery is especially successful but should be clearly viewed against a mortality of essentially 100% if these babies do not receive surgery. This seemingly very obvious point is important as is emphasises that surgery in the context of NEC is very much a marker of disease severity. Babies that respond to medical therapy alone are on the whole not as unwell as those that present for surgery. Conversely, a mortality of around a third for babies who otherwise would have a survival rate of over 90% indicates the devastating impact of NEC. As overall outcomes for neonates have improved beyond recognition, NEC still has a high mortality. The subgroups of smaller neonates reflect the same pattern as NEC confers a much higher mortality compared to equivalent neonates who do not contract the disease. The same can be said for the morbidity of NEC in the survivors.

'Surgical disease'—babies who present requiring surgical intervention—therefore is clearly a marker of severity. The clinical pathway for most of these babies is that when they become unwell, they are commenced on medical therapy and some will then progress to needing surgery. It would therefore be a logical conclusion that there is not a mortality from 'medical NEC' and the data that shows a difference between the outcomes for all-comers (both medically and surgically treated babies) is simply reflecting that the mortality is in a subset and thus the denominator is larger. This is not correct. There is a definite mortality among babies who never have surgery as well as those that do. Some of these neonates will be too unwell for transfer to a surgical unit. Some will be deemed too unwell for a laparotomy when they present and some will have multiple other issues as well as their NEC. Some of the babies who get NEC become overwhelmingly septic and succumb relatively quickly. One study of ELBW infants suggests a mortality of 26% for medical NEC babies and 40% for surgical disease. The difference is significant but there remains a mortality among those who did not have any surgical procedures. One UK study showed that more than 40% of infants whose death was attributed to NEC had not undergone surgery [9]. The cohort with NEC not having surgery is much larger so the relative risk is correspondingly much smaller but it is not true to say that the mortality is only found in the surgical group.

9.4 Neurodevelopmental Disability

The term 'neurodevelopment disability' (NDD) encompasses a wide range of problems. All babies born prematurely are at higher risk of NDD. NEC undoubtedly confers a high risk of disability. The exact mechanism of this is not understood but the outcome data is very clear that acquiring NEC has a detrimental effect on the developing brain. There is also probably a 'dosage effect' in that babies that are more unwell with NEC (i.e. those that require surgical intervention) have poorer outcomes than those who had NEC that was managed medically.

9.4.1 Definition of Neurodevelopmental Disability (NDD)

NDD is essentially an umbrella term. In most of the literature it is defined as the presence of one or more of the following: cerebral palsy; bilateral blindness; bilateral hearing loss (needing amplification) and low scores on the Bayley Scale of Infant and Toddler Development (BSID). The US Centre for Disease Control and Prevention (CDC) defines cerebral palsy as "a group of disorders that affect a person's ability to move and maintain balance and posture" [10]. It is important to note that this covers a very wide spectrum from milder cases who have some difficulty walking to the more severe who usually cannot walk and have associated intellectual disability and seizures.

Classifications of "mild," "moderate," or "severe" are often used in the literature although there is not a complete consensus on the criteria for each of these. The implications for NEC survivors are similarly very variable. Many will have little or no long-term sequelae but conversely others, more severely affected will need lifelong care and support.

9.4.2   The Bayley Scales of Infant and Toddler Development (BSID)

The first commercially available and therefore widely usable BSID was released in 1969. Named after their creator Nancy Bayley who spent 40 years researching infant development leading up to the publication of what is now known as *The Bayley Scale of Infant Development I* (BSID-I). BSID-II was released in 1994. The third version—now named *The Bayley Scale of Infant and Toddler Development* (BSID-III)—was published in 2006. The latest iteration (BSID-IV) was released in 2019. BSID-I assessed the development of infants and toddlers aged 3 to 28 months in two domains: motor and mental. BSID-II added a behaviour assessment and went from 1 month up to 42 months of age. BSID-III expanded this to five domains: cognition, motor, language, socio-emotional, and adaptive behaviour. BSID-IV retains these five domains. Because of the new versions being released the NEC literature has changed over time with the introduction of each version. Much of the recent literature has used BSID-III, whilst older literature will have measured development with BSID-II. Similarly in the future, BSID-IV will supersede BSID-III [11].

In most of the NEC literature 'severe NDD'—implying significant implications for daily living and long term morbidity—is defined as the presence of the disabilities listed above or below specific threshold scores on the BSID. Typically a mental development index (MDI) score or a psychomotor developmental index (PDI) score of less than 70 is used as the threshold. Both scores are normalised with a mean of 100 and a standard deviation of 16, so that 70 is approximately two standard deviations below the mean.

There are some important criticisms and limitations to BSID. Primarily that it takes 30–70 min to administer the test properly so it is labour intensive. The data for the normograms that underpins the tests are primarily based on US infants and therefore may have less applicability to other populations. There is some debate in the literature as to how accurately a particular BSID score at the age of two predicts long-term function. It continues to be an evolving and developing area but the need for long-term follow-up and assessment of children who were born prematurely is clear, so that they can get the support they need. It is also clear that infants who have NEC are far more likely to have NDD (by whichever means it is defined) than infants born at the same gestation who do not contract NEC.

9.4.3   Mechanisms

The developing brain is especially vulnerable to injury. It would be an exaggeration to state that the mechanism by which NEC causes NDD is fully understood. However there is a lot of indirect evidence from both human and animal studies.

Some authors postulate that NEC is a truly systemic disease and that the intestinal manifestation that is seen is essentially a symptom of systemic compromise. In this paradigm, effects on other organ systems are not remotely surprising. Conversely, there is a lot of evidence around the mechanisms of NEC itself that fit with it being a primary intestinal disease (albeit one that has systemic triggers) with systemic effects due to the large inflammatory response that NEC induces.

Periventricular leukomalacia (PVL) and severe intraventricular haemorrhage (IVH) can be demonstrated in premature infants by radiological imaging. These manifestations of central nervous system (CNS) injury in the preterm infant correlate with an increased risk of adverse neurodevelopmental outcome in the long term [12]. Both PVL and IVH are often seen in babies following an episode of NEC. Yoon et al. [13] compared post mortem specimens from infants with PVL with those from control infants without PVL. They demonstrated that affected infants had significantly increased staining of the inflammatory cytokines TNF-α, IL-1β and IL-6. This supports the idea that PVL could be a secondary effect of these systemic cytokines.

The large systemic inflammatory response to NEC is well established. Infants with NEC have a rise in multiple inflammatory cytokines. Therefore a working explanation of NDD secondary to NEC is that the systemic inflammatory response damages the developing brain [14]. There is also evidence that the intestinal microbiota changes associated with NEC affects the developing brain and could be an important mechanism in inducing brain injury [14]. Sometimes this injury is evident with increased rates of PVL and IVH but often the poorer neurodevelopmental outcomes are seen without PVL and/or IVH being demonstrated. This implies that PVL/IVH are 'visible' manifestations of brain injury but that injury may still be occurring even if they are not evident.

9.4.4   Rates of Severe NDD

The estimated rates of NDD following NEC vary significantly. Estimates range from 25% to over 60% [8]. Data from the biggest studies would put the true figure around 30%. The risk of NDD correlates with both prematurity and severity of illness: the most premature infants have higher rates of NDD and infants who require surgery for NEC have higher rates than those treated medically.

More recent work also shows the association between NDD and NEC in both the presence and absence of IVH. Culbreath et al. showed that having surgery for NEC was associated with an increased risk of NDD [15] and the risk was also correlated with the degree of IVH. In their series of nearly 6000 infants, 33.9% of ELBW babies who had surgery for NEC without IVH and survived to follow-up, had severe NDD (compared to only 17.6% of babies who did not contract NEC). In babies diagnosed with mild IVH in addition to needing surgery for NEC, the rate of severe NDD was 35.4% and 75% in babies with severe IVH. Babies with severe IVH without NEC had rates of severe NDD of over 50%. These data show that surgical NEC is an independent risk factor for NDD both with and without IVH but also that IVH is a good prognostic indicator in babies. It is not uncommon that cranial ultrasound reveals more severe IVH after infants have had surgery for NEC.

9.5   Intestinal Failure

9.5.1   Definitions of Intestinal Failure and Short Bowel Syndrome

There are various accepted definitions of intestinal failure (IF) but the following is probably the most useful in this context:

> Intestinal failure in children is as a reduction in functional intestine below that which is necessary for adequate digestion and absorption of fluid and nutrients required for healthy growth. [16]

Short bowel syndrome (SBS) is the term used when a congenital absence of intestine (i.e. due to an atresia or other in-utero event) or subsequent loss due to surgical resection, results in insufficient intestine for normal function. A key point about children is that they need to grow. Unlike an adult whereby fluid and nutrition are needed just to maintain haemostasis, children should be growing and developing. There is significant debate as to how much residue small bowel is enough to feed and grow. There is significant variation in how SBS is defined. One commonly used definition is that SBS is present when a child has less than 25% of the expected length of small bowel for their gestational age [17–19]. Especially in the context of NEC, this definition is useful as many of the babies undergo surgery and resection at a low gestational age.

Implicitly, a definition of SBS based on expected bowel length depends on having an accurate idea of what normal length for gestational age actually is. Unfortunately there is some variation is these figures. Struijs et al. (2009) [20] is widely cited as a basis for these estimates. They measured the length of small bowel found in 108 infants and children who underwent surgery for several different indications. More recently Bardwell et al. (2022) [21] used post-mortem studies from 131 foetuses and infants to estimate intestinal length. Stuijs's data showed a mean small bowel length of 70 cm for babies between 24 and 26 weeks gestation, rising to 160 cm at term and 240 cm at 6 months post term. Bardwell's data estimates mean small bowel length at 150 cm at 25 weeks and 300 cm at term. Whilst this large variation is disappointing and shows there is definitely more work to be done to establish meaningful nomograms, there is notable agreement that intestinal length will double from around 24 weeks to term. Consequentially the estimate of 25% of expected length has a wide variation between 20–40 cm at 25 weeks and 40–75 cm at term. Some of this discrepancy may be technical and simply reflect that measuring healthy intestine intra-operatively is different to measuring intestine post mortem. Although it seems unlikely that it is sufficient to explain the twofold difference in these datasets.

Arguably, the term *intestinal failure* (IF) is more useful than *short bowel syndrome* (SBS) and should be preferred. Children with the same amount of small bowel can have very different function. It is not so much a question of how much bowel an individual has, as how well the intestine they have functions. This is often encapsulated in the phrase 'functional short bowel' implying that the amount is theoretically sufficient but in practice the absorption of nutrients and fluid is actually inadequate. *Intestinal Failure* encompasses all of these situations. The problem with the definition of IF given above, is that it inevitably implies parental-nutrition dependence. This excludes some children who when feeding on a normal diet are unable to grow and develop normally. Some of these children will be managed by special feeds, different feeding strategies and medication. Restricting a definition of IF to those that are PN-dependent means these children who have significant healthcare needs as well are not captured in the data.

9.5.2   Necrotising Enterocolitis and Intestinal Failure

NEC is a leading cause of IF in children with between a quarter and third of cases of IF in children being attributed to NEC [22]. Other causes include volvulus, intestinal atresia, gastroschisis and total colonic Hirschsprung disease (with small bowel aganglionosis). Given that NEC surgery necessitates bowel resection of a variable amount (depending on the extent of the disease), it is unsurprising that NEC is responsible for a high proportion of IF in children. Even with little or no bowel resection, NEC is associated with poor feed tolerance for a variable amount of time. The majority of studies that report IF associated with NEC report parenteral nutrition (PN)-dependence at 90 days. This is a useful but incomplete measure. It is useful as it shows that 3 months after acute illness and surgery, many babies are still not able to feed and grow normally. Again this emphasises that NEC is an acute illness that can often have long-term (or even life-long) consequences. Conversely, it is not a sufficient way to encompass all of IF in NEC. Most babies still requiring PN at 3 months will achieve enteral autonomy. It is a very different health and societal burden to require PN after discharge than to be on it only whilst an infant in a neonatal unit.

By this measure (PN-dependence at 90 days) between 15% and 35% of infants who undergo surgery for NEC will have IF [8]. To some extent this range reflects that different studies looked at different populations: as with mortality and NDD, the smallest babies have the worst outcomes. The rate of PN dependence at 2 years post NEC is reported at around 6% [23]. This is consistent with other reports that show the majority of children with IF due to NEC will achieve enteral autonomy eventually. A single large study shows that by 72 months post diagnosis of IF, 60% of children will achieve enteral autonomy if the IF is secondary to NEC [22].

From a pragmatic, clinical perspective, whilst precise prognostication is difficult, there is a relatively clear pathway for these patients:

- Many babies after surgery for NEC will require parenteral nutrition.
- Around a fifth of these babies will still require PN after 90 days.
- Large (i.e. greater than 75%) resections imply a risk of short bowel syndrome.
- Whilst the length of residual bowel does correlate with function, it is not a perfect correlation and babies with the same length of bowel may have very different function.
- The majority of babies will achieve enteral autonomy, although some of these will be on PN for years.

9.5.3   Management of Intestinal Failure in Infants and Children

As noted above, IF in children is an inability to absorb sufficient nutrients and fluids for normal growth and development. IF is a complex disease and the severity of the malabsorption is determined by the length and quality of the remaining bowel [24].

A key concept in IF is *intestinal adaptation*. Intestinal adaptation is the process by which the residue gastrointestinal tract responds to the physiological needs of the individual [25, 26]. This is a process that takes place over months to years. The nature of the residual intestine is important. Much of the literature focuses simply on the length of small intestine. That suggests that the colon is unimportant which is not true. Similarly it has been known for some time that the presence of the ileo-caecal valve is a positive prognostic factor.

Aligned with the concept of adaptation is *intestinal rehabilitation*. The management of IF in children is complex and can only be done by a broad multidisciplinary team including paediatricians, paediatric surgeons, gastroenterology specialists, nutritionists, nurses and other professionals. The evidence shows that such a multidisciplinary approach focused on intestinal rehabilitation is associated with earlier weaning from PN, and improved survival [24]. Whilst PN is a vital part of the management of IF, it is not without its problems, notably central-line associated complications and progressive liver failure.

Intestinal adaptation occurs in response to significant bowel loss. In paediatric patients it begins shortly after the loss of intestinal length and continues for several years. In the initial stages, there is epithelial hyperplasia which includes lengthening of residual villi and deepening of the crypts. There is also proliferation of microvilli. This results in a very large increase in the intestinal surface area without any anatomical changes. However, anatomical changes also occur in the form of dilatation and elongation of the residual bowel [27]. The overall effect of this is that the intestine progressively gains functionality which in simplistic terms can be quantified by the reduced need for PN. A patient may initially require all of their nutrition from PN but over time the calorie (and other nutrient) requirement is increasingly met by enteral feeds.

As noted above, considering only small bowel length is overly simplistic. The ileum has greater adaptive capacity than the jejunum [24]. Moreover, the ileum is responsible for the absorption of vitamin B12 and bile salts. The enterohepatic circulation is important for effective digestion. Human metabolism produces bile salts in the liver which are then excreted in bile. These are reabsorbed in the terminal ileum whereby they pass back to the liver in the portal circulation and are secreted again in bile. This process is important not just because the bile salts are retained and reused by the body but because they undergo significant modification by the normal intestinal flora [28]. This biological modification of bile salts creates a much more diverse range of molecules which significantly enhances the function of the bile salts in digestion and intestinal health. Therefore loss of the terminal ileum implies a much narrower range of bile salts impairing digestion and absorption of nutrients. Resection of the caecum implies loss of the ileo-caecal valve (ICV). The clinical significance of this has been debated for some time but there is undoubtedly a correlation between retaining the ICV and better outcomes in intestinal failure [29]. Whether the ICV is itself important or simply a marker of terminal ileal resection continues to be a key subject of debate. At the very least it is plausible that both are true. For the reasons discussed, the retention of ileum—especially distal ileum—is important for adaptation and long-term intestinal function. The function of the ICV is thought to be twofold. It slows intestinal transit time thereby increasing mucosal surface contact of enteric contents and promoting nutrient absorption. It also plays a role in preventing small bowel intestinal bacterial overgrowth which is related to the reflux of colonic contents into the small bowel. Bacterial overgrowth results in a malabsorbative state causing diarrhoea and malnutrition [24].

Undoubtedly the colon is of less importance than the small intestine. However that is not to say it is unimportant. The main function of the large intestine is the reabsorption of water and hence patients who have lost their colon are at higher risk of dehydration. From a quality of life point of view, the frequency of stooling can be very high in a patient without a colon. More recently the role of glucagon-like peptide 2 (GLP-2) has become the subject of much study, especially with a view to its potential as a therapeutic agent. GLP-2 is an intestinal growth factor. A GLP-2 analogue has been shown to reduce PN dependence [30]. The mechanism of action is that is promotes intestinal adaptation. Physiologically, GLP-2 is produced in the terminal ileum and the ascending colon. The implication is that resection of the proximal colon may reduce the ability of the residual intestinal tract to adapt.

Parenteral nutrition is at the centre of the management of intestinal failure. Whilst the hope and aim is to achieve enteral autonomy, implicitly, most patients will require PN for some period of time. There are essentially three major life-threatening risks of PN. PN requires central venous access. The incidence of (central) catheter-related bloodstream infection is estimated at 1.3–10 per 1000 catheter days [31]. Patients with IF may have a central venous catheter for hundreds or thousands of days and PN is a very nutrient-rich medium that is conducive to bacterial growth. The risk is higher in patients under a year of age.

The second notable risk is hepatic failure. Intestinal failure-associated liver disease (IFALD) is a cholestatic disorder that develops in children receiving long-term

PN. The risk correlates with the length of time on PN. The development of IFLAD is multifactorial. Sepsis—usually secondary to central venous catheter usage—is a major risk factor. Convention lipids used in PN are plant based and are strongly associated with IFLAD. The mechanisms are complex but conventional lipids are proinflammatory. More recent practice has mostly replaced conventional lipid with SMOF. "SMOF" stands for soy, medium-chain triglyceride, olive and fish oils. Direct trial comparison data is quite limited [32] but the adoption into routine practice has anecdotally resulted in a notable reduction in hepatic dysfunction.

The third risk is central venous catheter-associated thrombosis. Rarely is the thrombosis itself of any direct clinical consequence. However the presence of thrombosis can make a vein unavailable for access. Thrombosis in multiple veins can make central access very difficult and thus is a leading indication for small-bowel transplantation in children [33]. Traditionally central lines were inserted with an open, 'cut-down' technique. Whilst few direct comparison trials have been conducted, the use of ultrasound guidance and a percutaneous approach results in the lowest reported rate of venous occlusion at only 3% [34]. This is particularly important in infants and children who may need central access for a prolonged period of time. A more recent small study in infants weighing less than 10 kg showed the rate of venous occlusion from a percutaneously inserted line to be less than half that of lines inserted with an open technique [35].

9.5.4   Management Considerations in Acute NEC

Intestinal failure is a foreseeable but not necessarily avoidable consequence of NEC. In an ideal world, surgical resection would be kept to a minimum. The correlation with extensive bowel resection and adverse outcome is clear cut. Similarly, retention of the terminal ileum, ileo-caecal valve and ascending colon are desirable. The nature of NEC surgery does not usually give the luxury of choice. Necrotic bowel necessitates resection. However, if a particular surgical approach resulted in less resection being needed this could be beneficial. Surgical strategies are discussed in more detail in Chap. 8, but one approach to acutely unwell infants is the use of laparostomy and a second-look laparotomy. A potential advantage of this approach is that it may be possible to resect intestine that is frankly necrotic whilst leaving behind intestine that may recover for a review at a second operation. No clear data exists, but it is possible that such an approach would result in more intestine being retained which could be important for the long term intestinal function.

A more straight-forward consideration is the approach to central venous access. In infants with significant intestinal resection, the long-term need for PN is predictable. Such babies will therefore need central venous access for a number of years. The data on percutaneous versus open approaches—whilst not totally conclusive—support a much lower rate of venous occlusion. This is a very strong argument for preferring the percutaneous approach in these patients to reduce the risk of them running out of central venous access in later years whilst they remain PN-dependent.

9.6 Other Morbidities

Infants born prematurely often have on-going healthcare needs throughout childhood and beyond. Babies who contract NEC have higher rates of requiring hospital admission in the first 2 years of life than comparable infants who did not contract NEC.

ELBW infants who have had NEC have a rehospitalisation rate approaching 40% in one study. In those who had surgery for NEC, it is over 50% [2]. The reasons for readmission include respiratory illness, nutritional needs (failure to thrive) and sepsis.

9.7 Overall Outcomes

The outcome data on NEC is stark. Whilst it is an acute illness that is often managed surgically, it is also a harbinger of life-long morbidity. NEC outcomes, should be taken in context. All babies born prematurely are at risk of mortality (significantly higher than the background rate of infant mortality) and of complications. However, a baby born today, 3 months premature has very good odds of surviving and a good chance of surviving without significant disability.

This is one of the great success stories of modern medicine: babies born prematurely without a congenital anomaly have good outcomes. This is not true if they contract NEC. Figure 9.1 illustrates this point. The data here is from babies with a birthweight of less 1000 g (ELBW) and therefore those with the highest risk of an adverse outcome. In this dataset (based on over 10,000 infants in the US), the overall survival for babies who did not contract NEC is approaching 90% with over 70% of them surviving without significant NDD. Survival (to 2 years of age) drops to 73% in those that had medically treated NEC and only 62% in those that had NEC requiring surgical intervention. This pattern in mirrored in the NDD data such that for a ELBW baby who has had surgery for NEC, the chance of survival without significant disability is around 39%—just over half that of an equivalent infant who did not contract NEC.

Intestinal failure after NEC is the other major long-term sequelae. Whilst babies who are discharged on PN have a very good chance of achieving enteral autonomy in childhood there are multiple adverse consequences of intestinal failure. This includes an effect on brain development. Probably, due to the fact that whilst modern PN is increasingly sophisticated, it is not as good as enteral feeding at providing complete nutrition. Overall children with IF have higher rates of NDD.

Ultimately, NEC remains a devastating disease with both a high mortality and significant morbidity for many of the survivors. Survivors may well have neurodevelopmental disability, intestinal failure or other medical needs. For many this will mean life-long adverse consequences. The data from literally hundreds of studies,

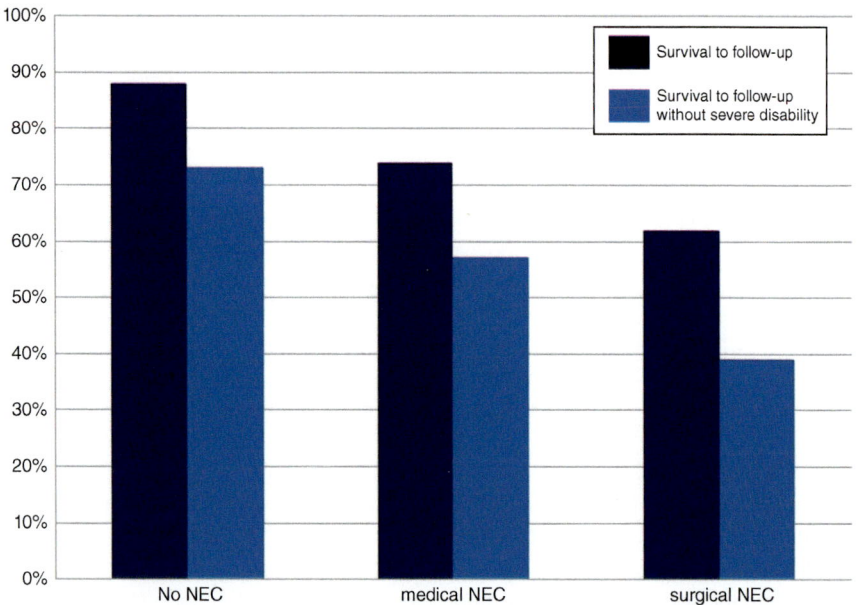

Fig. 9.1 Outcomes for ELBW with and without NEC (*based on* Fullerton et al. [2]). The majority of babies with a birthweight below 1000 g, who do not contract NEC, survive with nearly three quarters surviving without severe disability. This falls to less than two thirds surviving in the group that require surgery for NEC and less than 40% surviving without severe disability

show that effective preventative measures and better treatments for NEC are desperately needed. The next chapter is dedicated to the current state of the art of research aimed at finding better options for caring for infants at risk of NEC and how to better treat them when they do succumb.

References

1. Klerk D, van Varsseveld O, Offringa M, Modi N, Lacher M, Zani A, et al. Development of an international core outcome set for treatment trials in necrotizing enterocolitis—a study protocol. Trials. 2023;24(1):367. https://doi.org/10.1186/s13063-023-07413-x.
2. Fullerton BS, Hong CR, Velazco CS, Mercier CE, Morrow KA, Edwards EM, et al. Severe neurodevelopmental disability and healthcare needs among survivors of medical and surgical necrotizing enterocolitis: a prospective cohort study. J Pediatr Surg. 2017; https://doi.org/10.1016/j.jpedsurg.2017.10.029.
3. Fitzgibbons SC, Ching Y, Yu D, Carpenter J, Kenny M, Weldon C, et al. Mortality of necrotizing enterocolitis expressed by birth weight categories. J Pediatr Surg. 2009;44(6):1072–5.; ; discussion 5–6. https://doi.org/10.1016/j.jpedsurg.2009.02.013.
4. The United Nations Inter-agency Group for Child Mortality Estimation. Levels & trends in child mortality estimation report 2020. 2020. https://www.unicef.org/media/79371/file/UN-IGME-child-mortality-report-2020.pdf.pdf.

5. Janik J, Ein S, Mancer K. Intestinal stricture after necrotizing enterocolitis. J Pediatr Surg. 1981;16(4):438–43. https://doi.org/10.1016/s0022-3468(81)80002-4.

6. Gaudin A, Farnoux C, Bonnard A, Alison M, Maury L, Biran V, Baud O. Necrotizing enterocolitis (NEC) and the risk of intestinal stricture: the value of C-reactive protein. PLoS One. 2013;8(10):e76858. https://doi.org/10.1371/journal.pone.0076858.

7. Montalva L, Incerti F, Qoshe L, Haffreingue A, Marsac L, Frérot A, et al. Early laparoscopic-assisted surgery is associated with decreased post-operative inflammation and intestinal strictures in infants with necrotizing enterocolitis. J Pediatr Surg. 2023;58(4):708–14. https://doi.org/10.1016/j.jpedsurg.2022.11.007.

8. Jones IH, Hall NJ. Contemporary outcomes for infants with necrotizing enterocolitis-a systematic review. J Pediatr. 2020;220:86–92. https://doi.org/10.1016/j.jpeds.2019.11.011.

9. Battersby C, Longford N, Mandalia S, Costeloe K, Modi N. Incidence and enteral feed antecedents of severe neonatal necrotising enterocolitis across neonatal networks in England, 2012–13: a whole-population surveillance study. Lancet Gastroenterol Hepatol. 2017;2(1):43–51. https://doi.org/10.1016/s2468-1253(16)30117-0.

10. CDC. What is cerebral palsy? CDC. 2024. https://www.cdc.gov/ncbddd/cp/facts.html.

11. Balasundaram P, Avulakunta I. Bayley scales of infant and toddler development. Treasure Island: StatPearls Publishing; 2024.

12. Law J, Wood T, Gogcu S, Comstock B, Dighe M, Perez K, et al. Intracranial hemorrhage and 2-year neurodevelopmental outcomes in infants born extremely preterm. J Pediatr. 2021;238:124–134.e10. https://doi.org/10.1016/j.jpeds.2021.06.071.

13. Yoon B, Romero R, Kim C, Koo J, Choe G, Syn H, Chi J. High expression of tumor necrosis factor-alpha and interleukin-6 in periventricular leukomalacia. Am J Obstet Gynecol. 1997;177(2):406–11. https://doi.org/10.1016/s0002-9378(97)70206-0.

14. Lu J, Martin C, Claud E. Neurodevelopmental outcome of infants who develop necrotizing enterocolitis: the gut-brain axis. Semin Perinatol. 2023;47(1):151694. https://doi.org/10.1016/j.semperi.2022.151694.

15. Culbreath K, Keefe G, Nes E, Edwards E, Knell J, Morrow K, et al. Association between neurodevelopmental outcomes and concomitant presence of NEC and IVH in extremely low birth weight infants. J Perinatol. 2024;44(1):108–15. https://doi.org/10.1038/s41372-023-01780-8.

16. Barclay AR, Beattie LM, Weaver LT, Wilson DC. Systematic review: medical and nutritional interventions for the management of intestinal failure and its resultant complications in children. Aliment Pharmacol Ther. 2011;33(2):175–84. https://doi.org/10.1111/j.1365-2036.2010.04514.x.

17. Salvia G, Guarino A, Terrin G, Cascioli C, Paludetto R, Indrio F, et al. Neonatal onset intestinal failure: an Italian Multicenter Study. J Pediatr. 2008;153(5):674–6. https://doi.org/10.1016/j.jpeds.2008.05.017.

18. Wales P, de Silva N, Kim J, Lecce L, To T, Moore A. Neonatal short bowel syndrome: population-based estimates of incidence and mortality rates. J Pediatr Surg. 2004;39(5):690–5. https://doi.org/10.1016/j.jpedsurg.2004.01.036.

19. Grant D. Intestinal transplantation: 1997 report of the international registry. Intestinal Transplant Registry. Transplantation. 1999;67(7):1061–4. https://doi.org/10.1097/00007890-199904150-00021.

20. Struijs M, Diamond I, de Silva N, Wales P. Establishing norms for intestinal length in children. J Pediatr Surg. 2009;44(5):933–8. https://doi.org/10.1016/j.jpedsurg.2009.01.031.

21. Bardwell C, El Demellawy D, Oltean I, Murphy M, Agarwal A, Hamid J, et al. Establishing normal ranges for fetal and neonatal small and large intestinal lengths: results from a prospective postmortem study. World J Pediatr Surg. 2022;5(3):e000397. https://doi.org/10.1136/wjps-2021-000397.

22. Khan FA, Squires RH, Litman HJ, Balint J, Carter BA, Fisher JG, et al. Predictors of enteral autonomy in children with intestinal failure: a multicenter cohort study. J Pediatr. 2015;167(1):29–34.e1. https://doi.org/10.1016/j.jpeds.2015.03.040.

23. Sjoberg Bexelius T, Ahle M, Elfvin A, Bjorling O, Ludvigsson JF, Andersson RE. Intestinal failure after necrotising enterocolitis: incidence and risk factors in a Swedish population-based longitudinal study. BMJ Paediatr Open. 2018;2(1):e000316. https://doi.org/10.1136/bmjpo-2018-000316.
24. Caporilli C, Giannì G, Grassi F, Esposito S. An overview of short-bowel syndrome in pediatric patients: focus on clinical management and prevention of complications. Nutrients. 2023;15(10):2341. https://doi.org/10.3390/nu15102341.
25. Batra A, Keys S, Johnson M, Wheeler R, Beattie R. Epidemiology, management and outcome of ultrashort bowel syndrome in infancy. Arch Dis Child Fetal Neonatal Ed. 2017;102(6):F551–6. https://doi.org/10.1136/archdischild-2016-311765.
26. Thompson J, Rochling F, Weseman R, Mercer D. Current management of short bowel syndrome. Curr Probl Surg. 2012;49(2):52–115. https://doi.org/10.1067/j.cpsurg.2011.10.002.
27. Warner B. The pathogenesis of resection-associated intestinal adaptation. Cell Mol Gastroenterol Hepatol. 2016;2(4):429–38. https://doi.org/10.1016/j.jcmgh.2016.05.001.
28. Di Ciaula A, Garruti G, Lunardi Baccetto R, Molina-Molina E, Bonfrate L, Wang D, Portincasa P. Bile acid physiology. Ann Hepatol. 2017;16(Suppl. 1: s3-105):S4–S14. https://doi.org/10.5604/01.3001.0010.5493.
29. Goulet O, Baglin-Gobet S, Talbotec C, Fourcade L, Colomb V, Sauvat F, et al. Outcome and long-term growth after extensive small bowel resection in the neonatal period: a survey of 87 children. Eur J Pediatr Surg. 2005;15(2):95–101. https://doi.org/10.1055/s-2004-821214.
30. Overview. Teduglutide for treating short bowel syndrome. Guidance. NICE. 2024. https://www.nice.org.uk/guidance/ta804.
31. Fullerton B, Hong C, Jaksic T. Long-term outcomes of pediatric intestinal failure. Semin Pediatr Surg. 2017;26(5):328–35. https://doi.org/10.1053/j.sempedsurg.2017.09.006.
32. Diamond I, Grant R, Pencharz P, de Silva N, Feldman B, Fitzgerald P, et al. Preventing the progression of intestinal failure-associated liver disease in infants using a composite lipid emulsion: a pilot randomized controlled trial of SMOFlipid. JPEN J Parenter Enteral Nutr. 2017;41(5):866–77. https://doi.org/10.1177/0148607115626921.
33. Kaufman S, Avitzur Y, Beath S, Ceulemans L, Gondolesi G, Mazariegos G, Pironi L. New insights into the indications for intestinal transplantation: consensus in the year 2019. Transplantation. 2020;104(5):937–46. https://doi.org/10.1097/TP.0000000000003065.
34. Wragg R, Blundell S, Bader M, Sharif B, Bennett J, Jester I, et al. Patency of neck veins following ultrasound-guided percutaneous Hickman line insertion. Pediatr Surg Int. 2014;30(3):301–4. https://doi.org/10.1007/s00383-013-3416-3.
35. Vierboom L, Darani A, Langusch C, Soundappan S, Karpelowsky J. Tunnelled central venous access devices in small children: a comparison of open vs. ultrasound-guided percutaneous insertion in children weighing ten kilograms or less. J Pediatr Surg. 2018;53(9):1832–8. https://doi.org/10.1016/j.jpedsurg.2018.03.025.

Chapter 10
Novel and Potential Future Treatments

Contents

Abstract NEC is a devastating disease with significant mortality and life-long morbidity for the survivors. Current therapies are clearly inadequate and there is a clear need for better treatments.

Within the basic science realm there are a number of potential treatments which could be translated to clinical practice. There is a need for research to develop these into viable treatments.

Potential future treatments include: breast-milk derived components like lactoferrin; stem-cell-based therapies; microbiota transplant; immunotherapy; controlled hypothermia and remote ischaemic conditioning.

The incredible progress in neonatal care in general over the past few decades has not been matched by progress in NEC treatments. These interventions show the potential for future therapies and how currently the translation to practical and effective clinical treatments is sadly lacking.

© The Author(s), under exclusive license to Springer Nature
Switzerland AG 2024
I. Jones, *Necrotising Enterocolitis in Clinical Practice*, In Clinical Practice,
https://doi.org/10.1007/978-3-031-64148-0_10

Keywords NEC novel treatments · Future treatments for NEC · Innovative approaches to NEC management · Emerging therapies for NEC · Experimental treatments for NEC · Targeted therapies for NEC · Stem cell therapy for NEC Gene therapy for NEC · Immunomodulatory treatments for NEC · Nanotechnology in NEC treatment · Pharmacological interventions for NEC · Biomarker-guided therapy for NEC · Precision medicine in NEC management · Microbiota-based therapies for NEC · Epigenetic therapies for NEC · Nutraceuticals for NEC prevention and treatment · Cell-based therapies for NEC · Tissue engineering approaches for NEC · Artificial intelligence in NEC management · Clinical trials for novel NEC treatments

10.1 Introduction

This book is designed to set out the state of the art for Necrotising enterocolitis. Previous chapters have reviewed the history of the disease and how we got to where we are today. The outcomes for NEC in the twenty-first century remain poor. Around a quarter of babies will die and a large proportion of the survivors are left with life-long disease and disability [1]. The outcomes are discussed in detail in Chap. 9, but sadly overall they remain poor for many of the babies who contract NEC.

Chapter 6 discusses the preventative measures that are currently available for NEC. It is encouraging that antenatal corticosteroids have been shown to be beneficial and there is a likely to be a role for probiotic administration. However, it remains true to say that the incidence of NEC has not fallen significantly and some studies suggest rising rates due to the increased survival of extremely premature infants and therefore an increase in the at-risk population.

The stark fact is that we need new better therapies for NEC that can both prevent the disease and treat it more effectively and therefore improve outcomes. The purpose of this chapter is to describe research that exists that offers the hope of such therapies and their potential to improve outcomes.

It is always challenging bringing putative therapies through from basic science to clinical application, but there are particular challenges in researching diseases like NEC. NEC is a rare disease. This means that there is less research interest and funding than in some areas. One of the impacts of this is that there is simply less basic science research being done than is needed to develop new therapies. It also means that the studies needed for translation to clinical practice are few and far between.

As well as affecting research interest and funding, the rarity of a disease like NEC has practical implications on research. Most of the kind of studies needed, require broad collaborations between multiple centres. It is often necessary to collaborate internationally in order to recruit the kind of numbers of patients that are needed to perform the type of clinical studies that are needed.

Added to these factors are the specific challenges of research in children—especially infants. For very good reasons, ethical approval of studies in these patients are rigorous. All of these challenges must be acknowledge and go some way to explain why NEC outcomes have not improved. However these are challenges and should not be barriers to research. Two important counterpoints here is the way that paediatric oncological outcomes have changed in recent decades and neonatal outcomes overall have improved dramatically. The outstanding improvement in survival in extremely premature babies shows what is possible in this area (Fig. 2.1). Moreover, paediatric oncology via groups like SIOP (The International Society of Paediatric Oncology) [2] show how effective international collaboration can be at improving outcomes.

The following sections describe some potential therapies that offer the hope of much better outcomes for babies with NEC in the future. Theoretically, at least, some of these could be translated to clinical practice relatively quickly if the efficacy in real-world practice can be demonstrated.

10.2   Breast Milk Components

The pathophysiology of NEC is discussed in detail in Chap. 5 and the role of breast milk versus formula feeds in Sect. 5.3. Formula feeds do confer a higher risk of NEC and partly this is due to the composition of the feed being pro-inflammatory and increased metabolic demand on the intestine (relative to breast milk feeds). However, the evidence also shows that breast milk contains multiple protective factors such as maternal IgA antibodies. Two other breast milk components, lactoferrin and oligosaccharides are of particular interest as they have the potential to be useful in practice [3].

10.2.1   Lactoferrin

Lactoferrin is the most abundant protein in colostrum. It has proven anti-inflammatory properties, mediated by its inhibition of IL-6 and TNF-α. Lactoferrin also increases cell turnover and therefore promotes the intestine's reparative capability and reduces apoptosis. A clinic trial protocol for the use of Lactoferrin to prevent sepsis including NEC has been published [4].

10.2.2   Oligosaccharide

The role of Toll-like receptor 4 (TLR4) in the pathogenesis of NEC is discussed in Sect. 5.5.1. TLR4 is one of a class of molecules that binds to bacterial antigens and as a consequence triggers an inflammatory response. This is part of the innate immune system's response to bacterial infection. In simplistic terms, NEC pathophysiology is, in part, an exaggerated inflammatory response, mediated by TLR4

[5]. Oligosaccharides in breast milk protect the intestine by inhibiting TLR4 expression [3]. Again, the potential for use of oligosaccharides is clear but as yet there are no studies that show it is effective clinically.

10.3 Stem Cell Therapy

Stem cells are the subject of research interest in countless diseases and NEC is no exception. Stem cells are a key part of the biology of all multicellular organisms. In simplistic terms, the early embryo is made up of only stem cells that will differentiate into different cell types. Differentiation is a multistep process: Pluripotent stem cells are capable of becoming multiple cell types. They differentiate into tissue specific stem cells which then further differentiate into functional cells that make up functioning organs. Stem cells, by definition have the ability to self-renew and to differentiate into various functioning cells in order to effect healing. It is this potential for healing that makes them so appealing as a potential therapy for such a broad spectrum of human disease.

Mesenchymal stem cells (MSCs) can be obtained from various sources and are able to differentiate into multiple cell lineages. Whilst not truly totipotent (able to become any cell type) like embryo-derived cells, they have a remarkable ability to form multiple different cell types and can be harvested from the same individual. Therefore from both an ethical and practical perspective, MSCs are the most promising avenue of research, with the simplest pathway of translation to clinical use.

10.3.1 Bone Marrow-Derived Mesenchymal Stem Cells

In animal experiments, bone-marrow derived MSCs have been administered both intraperitoneally and intravenously. The results show a reduction in inflammation and improved tissue regeneration in the model from both methods of administration [3]. Indeed, exosomes (nanovesicles containing RNA, DNA and protein) from MSCs can both prevent and treat NEC in an animal model [6]. This shows the potential of MSCs. They promote intestinal healing in a way that could be clinically effective for both prevention of NEC and treatment.

10.3.2 Amniotic Fluid Derived Mesenchymal Stem Cells

Amniotic fluid derived MSCs can be harvested by amniocentesis and caesarean section. They are therefore easier to collect and show similar effectiveness to MSCs derived from other sources [3, 6].

10.3.3 Translation of Stem Cell Therapy to Clinical Practice?

Results like these are very promising. However, here, at what is still very much an experimental stage, is where the research stalls, and there are currently no clinical trials in this area [3]. The challenges are significant but not necessarily insurmountable. Ethical concerns about stem cells are generally avoided by using MSCs rather than embryologically-derived cells. There is likely to be a risk of tumorigenesis from the use of MSCs but the use of exomes may avoid this risk. Although the safety profile does need to be established. From a technical perspective though, exosome production still needs further development, it is not yet at a stage where it could be used clinically, even if a therapeutic protocol existed. The potential here is huge and the early work shows that MSCs undoubtedly could be a very effective therapy but they remain a very long way from being available in routine clinical practice.

10.4 Faecal Microbiota Transplantation

Disruption of the normal development of the intestinal microbiome is undoubtedly part of the pathophysiology of NEC (see Sect. 5.4). Therefore, as with the clinical use of probiotics, an intervention that 'normalises' the microbiome is likely to be beneficial. The transplantation of faecal matter has been used to treat *Clostridium defficile* infection [7] and could be applied to NEC treatment and especially prevention.

   Animal studies in piglets have shown that faecal transplantation is possible and has beneficial effects. However there are unquestionably safety concerns as there is a need to screen the donors for potential pathogenic organisms which may be passed on and currently there is no practical way to do so that could be used in the clinical setting [8].

   Better understanding of the neonatal biome may lead to an effective therapeutic strategy but at present it remains very much a theoretical therapy rather than one that could be used.

10.5 Immunotherapy

NEC is an immune disease in the sense that one part of the pathogenesis is a significant inflammatory response (See Sect. 5.5). The preterm intestine has an exaggerated inflammatory response and therefore modulating the innate immune system, to dampen inflammation is a logical target for NEC therapy.

   Various molecules have been proposed as potential pharmaceutical agents in NEC, including Lithcholic acid, glycyrrhizin and Interleuking-1 receptor-associated kinase inhibitors [3, 9–11].

Each of these agents are designed to suppress the TLR4 mediated pathway of inflammation. The role of TLR4 is discussed in Sect. 5.5.1. The Pregnane X receptor (PXR) suppresses the activity of TLR4. PXR-knockout mice have a more severe disease phenotype. Lithocholic acid is an agonist of PXR and thus reduces TLR-4 levels and has been shown to be effective in an animal model. Similarly, glycyrrhizin suppresses TLR-4 and the downstream NF-κβ signalling pathway. Interleukin-1 receptor-associated kinase inhibitors (IRAK—inhibitors) act by suppressing IL-1-induced expression of TLR-4. These agents and approaches are very much at the basic-science stage only [12]. The potential for an agent to act on the TLR-4 pro-inflammatory pathway is clear but that is a very long way from having a clinically available drug. The short and long term effects, bioavailability, mode of delivery and method of production, of a putative pharmaceutical agent would all need to be established before it could considered for clinical use.

10.6 Therapeutic Hypothermia

Therapeutic hypothermia is well-established for the treatment of hypoxic ischaemic encephalopathy (HIE) in infants who suffer birth asphyxia. A Cochrane review published in 2013 recommended its use in term and late pre-term infants with HIE [13]. Clinical and experimental studies showed that neural death after an hypoxic insult occurs in two phases, the second phase beginning after about 6 h [14]. The mechanisms include hyperaemia, cytotoxic oedema, mitochondrial failure, and free radical damage but importantly the concept of 'secondary energy failure' has been shown to be predictive of outcome [15]. This later phase is therefore theoretically amenable to intervention by lowering the metabolic demand on the cells by cooling to 32–34 °C. Therapeutic mild hypothermia reduces the composite outcome of neurodevelopmental disability and death in infants with birth asphyxia by 25% [13]. Given that NEC is also an ischaemia-reperfusion disease, it is also potentially amenable to a similar intervention.

Animal model studies show that whole body hypothermia (maintaining body temperature at 31–32 °C) reduces intestinal damage [16]. It has also been shown that the systemic effects that result in damage to other organs can be ameliorated by hypothermia [17]. A pilot study in human neonates has shown that it is practical and safe to cool infants with NEC for 48 h [18]. However, it is a complex, time consuming and cumbersome intervention. This might go some way to explain why the research into hypothermia for NEC has stalled for over a decade.

However, more recently there has been renewed interest in this area. A non-randomised study published by Gonçalves-Ferri et al. in 2021 with 43 infants showed that cooling infants with a diagnosis of NEC (Bell stage II or III) for 48 h reduced the risk of perforation, the need for surgery and was associated with a lower mortality [19]. Importantly they describe their methodology as 'low-technology' suggesting that it is an intervention that could be more widely used. At the time of writing this is still a long way from being widely accepted, and the evidence is limited. However these results do suggest this is an area worthy of more attention.

10.7   Remote Ischaemic Conditioning

There is currently a lot of interest in remote ischaemic conditioning (RIC) as a potential therapy for NEC. Not least because it could be used as both a treatment and as a means of preventing NEC. A Phase I (Safety and efficacy) study has been completed with RIC that showed it would be practical to use in the clinical setting with no evidence of a detrimental effect [20]. A Phase II trial protocol has also been published [21].

10.7.1   Ischaemic Conditioning

The phenomenon of ischaemic conditioning was first discovered by Murry et al. in 1986 [22]. They were using dog hearts to investigate the nature of ischaemia-reperfusion injury (IRI). IRI is the pathological mechanism of multiple disease processes, most notably coronary heart disease and (ischaemic) stroke. IRI means that an organ or tissue suffers the loss of an adequate blood supply for a period of time (ischaemia), followed by the restoration of the blood supply (reperfusion) which results in significant tissue or organ damage [23]. The loss of an adequate blood supply is implicitly a non-sustainable state for a prolonged period of time. However, the paradox is that with short periods of ischaemia (such that the tissue survives), the majority of the damage is done during the reperfusion phase [24]. During reperfusion there is the generation of oxidants, calcium overload, endothelial dysfunction and a pronounced inflammatory response.

Murry's ground-breaking work showed that if the heart was 'conditioned' to an ischaemic state prior to an infarction, the tissue was protected against the IRI insult such that there was a massive reduction in the injury. Their protocol involved operating on anesthetised dogs who had an arterial clip applied to the left circumflex artery. A classical infarction was induced by occluding this artery for 40 min and then allowing it to reperfuse. The hearts were harvested and examined 4 days later. Experimental animals had four cycles of 5 min occlusion, followed by 5 min reperfusion, prior to the 40 min infarction. This simple expedient reduced the infarct size by 75%.

Zhou et al. subsequently showed that conditioning could also be protective if applied after the initial ischaemic insult. This is known as post conditioning [25]. Whilst biologically interesting, this phenomenon is of little clinical use. However the discovery of *remote conditioning* offers the tantalising prospect that it may be possible to make use of these pathways in clinical practice. *Remote* ischaemic conditioning (RIC) was discovered when it was shown that the conditioning stimulus could be applied to one organ or tissue and yet the protective effect is seen in every other organ as well. The most useful breakthrough from a clinical perspective was when it was shown that skeletal muscle could be the tissue that underwent conditioning which resulted in a protective effect. This is so useful from a practical perspective because skeletal muscle can be conditioned in a non-invasive way by simply inflating a blood pressure cuff on a limb above systolic pressure for a few minutes and then releasing it for a few minutes to provide the cycles of ischaemia and reperfusion [26].

The concept of RIC is to use cycles of a short, non-injurious ischaemic stimulus to produce a global protective effect.

Figure 10.1 shows a simplified schematic of how remote ischaemic conditioning works. Short cycles of a few minutes of ischaemia and reperfusion can be achieved in a limb by inflating a blood pressure cuff above systolic pressure and then releasing the pressure. This causes the skeletal muscle to release various factors which 'condition' other organs to be more resistant to an ischaemic insult.

Since the discovery of the phenomenon of RIC, multiple detailed studies have helped to develop an understanding of how this conditioning is transmitted from the conditioned tissue/organ to the rest of the body. The neuronal pathway has been demonstrated in a variety of ways, including by exogenous administration of neurotransmitters which mimics the protective effect of RIC in experimental models [27]. It has been demonstrated that a blood-born component is part of the

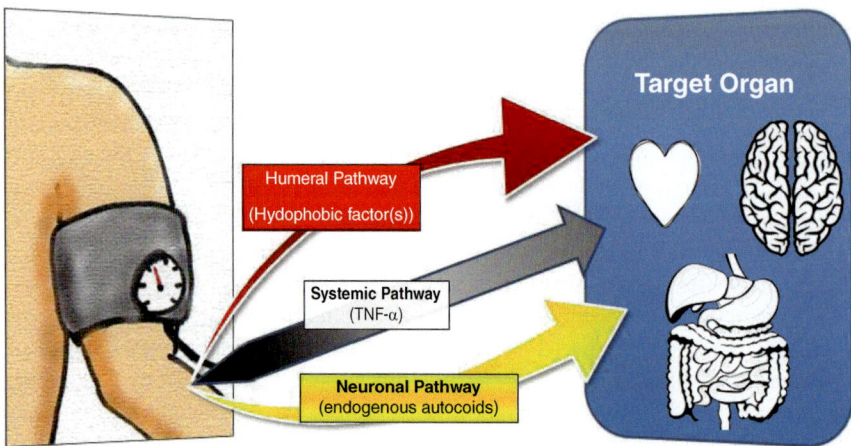

Fig. 10.1 Remote ischaemic conditioning provides a global protective effect by at least three separate, related pathways; humeral, systemic and neuronal

conduction of RIC by taking blood from a conditioned heart and administering it to naïve heart. This showed the same protective effect as conditioning the heart directly [28]. Several studies have shown that following RIC, circulating levels of multiple pro-inflammatory cytokines are reduced, including IL-10, IL-6 and TNF-α [29].

10.7.2   Failure of RIC Translation in Other Diseases

Murry's original work on ischaemic conditioning was in the heart. Since then, the majority of research interest has been in the context of cardiac disease. Whilst RIC has been found to be effective in every organ and species in which it has been investigated, the majority of the focus has been on cardiac disease. This is not surprising;, coronary artery disease is a leading cause of mortality and morbidity worldwide. The potential for an effective therapy in this area is massive. However, clinical studies have failed to demonstrate a benefit in human patients in most areas where it has been studied [30, 31]. This is not universally true, there are some areas where a benefit in humans has been demonstrated, including renal transplant [32]. However, in general, very promising results in animal studies has not translated into effective clinical treatments.

In an excellent review, McCafferty et al. [31] examined how comorbidities attenuate the effects of RIC, essentially trying to answer the question of why the consistent, dramatic results in animal studies have not translated to human medicine. They note that the participants in animal studies are often juvenile, of the same age with no comorbidities, as well as inbred, kept in the same environment and fed with the same diet. The point being that there are significant biological differences between the animals used in these studies and human patients with coronary artery disease, stroke or any other of the myriad of IRI conditions where RIC has shown promise. There is a lot of detailed data which shows how many of the comorbidities that are essentially ubiquitous in the human patients who might benefit from RIC, reduce the effectiveness of RIC [31].

NEC is a very different paradigm: The patients are juvenile, of the same age, kept in the same environment and lacking the comorbidities seen in adults. Conversely, NEC is not just an IRI disease, it is a complex, multifactorial process that ultimate results in necrosis. However, more recent work on RIC shows that there is a lot of cross-over between what could be termed 'anti-IRI pathways' and anti-inflammatory pathways. It is well established that RIC counteracts IRI but increasingly it appears to be a very effective anti-inflammatory intervention as well [33]. It has been shown that RIC activates anti-inflammatory pathways in the intestine, including in the intestine exposed to IRI [34]. Some of the animal work that demonstrates the potential for RIC in NEC is explored in the next section.

10.7.3   Animal Studies on RIC for NEC

Koike et al. [35] used a neonatal mouse gavage model of NEC. This involves feeding the mouse pups with a hyperosmolar formula with lipopolysaccharide and a hypoxic shock which induces and NEC-like illness in the pups. These animals are formula fed from birth and typically, this model produces 'NEC' with significant intestinal injury from around day 7 of life. They demonstrated that if the animals undergo RIC on day 5 or 6, the severity of disease seen is significantly reduced. One of the mechanism here is that RIC is improving the intestinal microcirculation [35].

Parallel work, using a model of NEC based on intestinal IRI shows similar, dramatic results. This model produces a profound injury to the small intestine. Nearly 90% of the exposed intestine will typically show evidence of injury. This is reduced to less than 50% in animals who had RIC prior to injury [36]. Microscopic analysis of the effected intestine shows a similar dramatic effect; animals who have RIC prior to injury have a much less severe injury. These results are shown in Fig. 10.2.

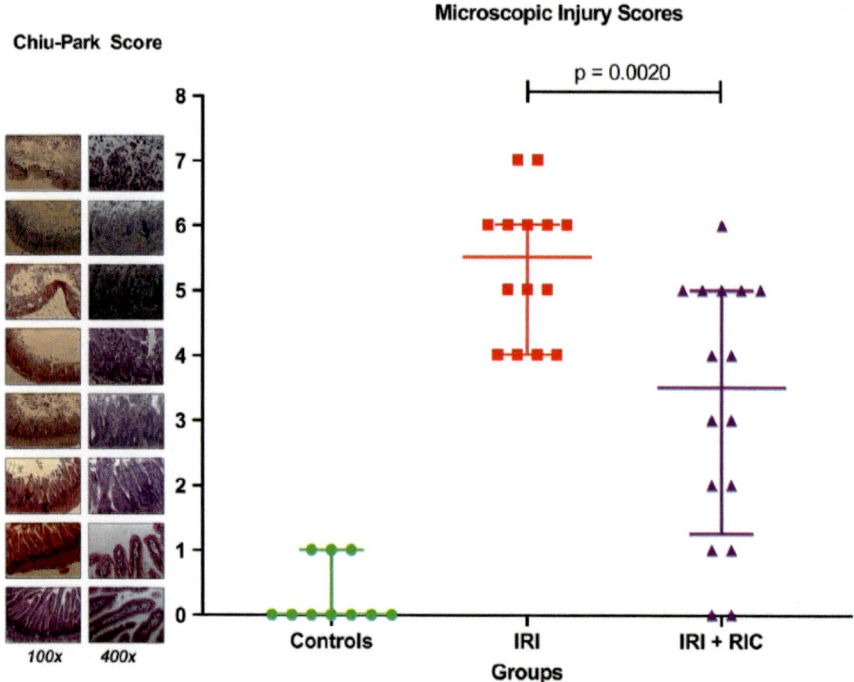

Fig. 10.2 Remote ischaemic conditioning significantly attenuates the intestinal injury of NEC in a rat model. The Chiu-Park scoring system is a validated system for analyses the severity of intestinal injury

The same study showed that RIC resulted in reduced neutrophil activity. Moreover there is a prolonged effect with RIC given 48 h prior to injury providing a protection and a dose-effect with animals that have RIC both 48 h and immediately prior to injury having the greatest benefit in terms of the severity of intestinal injury. RIC also has the potential to be used to prevent NEC as well as to treat it.

10.7.4   Potential for RIC in Preventing and Treating NEC

These studies show the potential for RIC in the intestine. If a similar effect is replicated in the gut of human neonates with evolving NEC, it is likely to make a measurable difference to their clinical course. The anti-inflammatory effect of RIC is also encouraging as it implies that RIC could counteract NEC at multiple stages in the pathogenesis and not just the most severe cases. Moreover, the trials of RIC in children undergoing cardiac surgery, along with the early trials of RIC for NEC support the notion that it can be safely delivered to preterm neonates.

10.8   Conclusion

There is no debate that NEC needs new therapies. The history of neonatal care is one of incredible success overall which shows what could be possible. And yet, NEC outcomes have lagged behind and remain mostly unchanged over several years. Time will tell, but future publications on NEC surely must be able to speak about new and more effective treatments. There is much to hope for in terms of reducing the incidence of NEC and seeing many more of the babies affected surviving and surviving without long-term consequences. The various putative therapies discussed here all have the potential. It may well be the case that a combination of interventions is the most effective way to both prevent and treat NEC. Some of these interventions are much closer to being translated to clinical practice than others. Some of these (and other) potential therapies may not work in clinical practice but it is only by developing them further and carrying out the necessary studies that this will become clear. It seems unlikely that all of them would fail if developed properly for clinical use. The key question and challenge for researchers in NEC is to ensure that potential therapies are discarded only if they are not applicable to the bedside.

Outcomes are not good enough for NEC. Which of these areas of research will yield the best results cannot be known, but the need to take on the challenge of developing new therapies for NEC, whilst great is an exciting one; there are many potential areas which might make this vital difference.

References

1. Jones IH, Hall NJ. Contemporary outcomes for infants with necrotizing enterocolitis—a systematic review. J Pediatr. 2020;220:86–92. https://doi.org/10.1016/j.jpeds.2019.11.011.
2. About | SIOP. 2024. https://siop-online.org/about/.
3. Wu H, Guo K, Zhuo Z, Zeng R, Luo Y, Yang Q, et al. Current therapy option for necrotizing enterocolitis: practicalities and challenge. Front Pediatr. 2022;10:954735. https://doi.org/10.3389/fped.2022.954735.
4. Bovine lactoferrin and neonatal survival in low birth weight babies. 2024. https://clinicaltrials.gov/study/NCT03431558.
5. Leaphart CL, Cavallo J, Gribar SC, Cetin S, Li J, Branca MF, et al. A critical role for TLR4 in the pathogenesis of necrotizing enterocolitis by modulating intestinal injury and repair. J Immunol. 2007;179(7):4808–20.
6. McCulloh C, Olson J, Wang Y, Zhou Y, Tengberg N, Deshpande S, Besner G. Treatment of experimental necrotizing enterocolitis with stem cell-derived exosomes. J Pediatr Surg. 2018;53(6):1215–20. https://doi.org/10.1016/j.jpedsurg.2018.02.086.
7. Kelly C, Khoruts A, Staley C, Sadowsky M, Abd M, Alani M, et al. Effect of fecal microbiota transplantation on recurrence in multiply recurrent clostridium difficile infection: a randomized trial. Ann Intern Med. 2016;165(9):609–16. https://doi.org/10.7326/M16-0271.
8. Brunse A, Martin L, Rasmussen T, Christensen L, Skovsted C, Wiese M, et al. Effect of fecal microbiota transplantation route of administration on gut colonization and host response in preterm pigs. ISME J. 2019;13(3):720–33. https://doi.org/10.1038/s41396-018-0301-z.
9. Huang K, Mukherjee S, DesMarais V, Albanese J, Rafti E, Draghi IA, et al. Targeting the PXR-TLR4 signaling pathway to reduce intestinal inflammation in an experimental model of necrotizing enterocolitis. Pediatr Res. 2018;83(5):1031–40. https://doi.org/10.1038/pr.2018.14.
10. Hou Y, Lu X, Zhang Y. IRAK inhibitor protects the intestinal tract of necrotizing enterocolitis by inhibiting the toll-like receptor (TLR) inflammatory signaling pathway in rats. Med Sci Monit. 2018;24:3366–73. https://doi.org/10.12659/MSM.910327.
11. Dai S, Sodhi C, Cetin S, Richardson W, Branca M, Neal M, et al. Extracellular high mobility group box-1 (HMGB1) inhibits enterocyte migration via activation of Toll-like receptor-4 and increased cell-matrix adhesiveness. J Biol Chem. 2010;285(7):4995–5002. https://doi.org/10.1074/jbc.M109.067454.
12. Ganji N, Li B, Lee C, Filler R, Pierro A. Necrotizing enterocolitis: state of the art in translating experimental research to the bedside. Eur J Pediatr Surg. 2019;29(4):352–60. https://doi.org/10.1055/s-0039-1693994.
13. Jacobs S, Berg M, Hunt R, Tarnow-Mordi W, Inder T, Davis P. Cooling for newborns with hypoxic ischaemic encephalopathy. Cochrane Database Syst Rev. 2013;2013(1):CD003311. https://doi.org/10.1002/14651858.CD003311.pub3.
14. Williams C, Gunn A, Gluckman P. Time course of intracellular edema and epileptiform activity following prenatal cerebral ischemia in sheep. Stroke. 1991;22(4):516–21. https://doi.org/10.1161/01.str.22.4.516.
15. Roth S, Baudin J, Cady E, Johal K, Townsend J, Wyatt J, et al. Relation of deranged neonatal cerebral oxidative metabolism with neurodevelopmental outcome and head circumference at 4 years. Dev Med Child Neurol. 1997;39(11):718–25. https://doi.org/10.1111/j.1469-8749.1997.tb07372.x.
16. Vejchapipat P, Proctor E, Ramsay A, Petros A, Gadian DG, Spitz L, Pierro A. Intestinal energy metabolism after ischemia-reperfusion: effects of moderate hypothermia and perfluorocarbons. J Pediatr Surg. 2002;37(5):786–90. https://doi.org/10.1053/jpsu.2002.32288.
17. Vinardi S, Pierro A, Parkinson EJ, Vejchapipat P, Stefanutti G, Spitz L, Eaton S. Hypothermia throughout intestinal ischaemia-reperfusion injury attenuates lung neutrophil infiltration. J Pediatr Surg. 2003;38(1):88–91. https://doi.org/10.1053/jpsu.2003.50017.

18. Hall N, Eaton S, Peters M, Hiorns M, Alexander N, Azzopardi D, Pierro A. Mild controlled hypothermia in preterm neonates with advanced necrotizing enterocolitis. Pediatrics. 2010;125(2):e300-8. https://doi.org/10.1542/peds.2008-3211.
19. Gonçalves-Ferri W, Ferreira C, Couto L, Souza T, de Castro PT, Carmona F, et al. Low technology, mild controlled hypothermia for necrotizing enterocolitis treatment: an initiative to improve healthcare to preterm neonates. Eur J Pediatr. 2021;180(10):3161–70. https://doi.org/10.1007/s00431-021-04014-1.
20. Zozaya C, Ganji N, Li B, Janssen L, Lee C, Koike Y, et al. Remote ischaemic conditioning in necrotising enterocolitis: a phase I feasibility and safety study. Arch Dis Child Fetal Neonatal Ed. 2023;108(1):69–76. https://doi.org/10.1136/archdischild-2022-324174.
21. Ganji N, Li B, Ahmad I, Daneman A, Deshpande P, Dhar V, et al. Remote ischemic conditioning in necrotizing enterocolitis: study protocol of a multi-center phase II feasibility randomized controlled trial. Pediatr Surg Int. 2022;38(5):679–94. https://doi.org/10.1007/s00383-022-05095-1.
22. Murry CE, Jennings RB, Reimer KA. Preconditioning with ischemia: a delay of lethal cell injury in ischemic myocardium. Circulation. 1986;74(5):1124–36.
23. Kalogeris T, Baines CP, Krenz M, Korthuis RJ. Cell biology of ischemia/reperfusion injury. Int Rev Cell Mol Biol. 2012;298:229–317. https://doi.org/10.1016/b978-0-12-394309-5.00006-7.
24. Jennings RB, Sommers HM, Smyth GA, Flack HA, Linn H. Myocardial necrosis induced by temporary occlusion of a coronary artery in the dog. Arch Pathol. 1960;70:68–78.
25. Zhao ZQ, Corvera JS, Halkos ME, Kerendi F, Wang NP, Guyton RA, Vinten-Johansen J. Inhibition of myocardial injury by ischemic postconditioning during reperfusion: comparison with ischemic preconditioning. Am J Physiol Heart Circ Physiol. 2003;285(2):H579–88. https://doi.org/10.1152/ajpheart.01064.2002.
26. Kristiansen SB, Henning O, Kharbanda RK, Nielsen-Kudsk JE, Schmidt MR, Redington AN, et al. Remote preconditioning reduces ischemic injury in the explanted heart by a KATP channel-dependent mechanism. Am J Physiol Heart Circ Physiol. 2005;288(3):H1252–6. https://doi.org/10.1152/ajpheart.00207.2004.
27. Heusch G. Molecular basis of cardioprotection: signal transduction in ischemic pre-, post-, and remote conditioning. Circ Res. 2015;116(4):674–99. https://doi.org/10.1161/CIRCRESAHA.116.305348.
28. Dickson EW, Reinhardt CP, Renzi FP, Becker RC, Porcaro WA, Heard SO. Ischemic preconditioning may be transferable via whole blood transfusion: preliminary evidence. J Thromb Thrombolysis. 1999;8(2):123–9.
29. Peralta C, Fernandez L, Panes J, Prats N, Sans M, Pique JM, et al. Preconditioning protects against systemic disorders associated with hepatic ischemia-reperfusion through blockade of tumor necrosis factor-induced P-selectin up-regulation in the rat. Hepatology (Baltimore, Md). 2001;33(1):100–13. https://doi.org/10.1053/jhep.2001.20529.
30. Benstoem C, Stoppe C, Liakopoulos OJ, Ney J, Hasenclever D, Meybohm P, Goetzenich A. Remote ischaemic preconditioning for coronary artery bypass grafting (with or without valve surgery). Cochrane Database Syst Rev. 2017;5:CD011719. https://doi.org/10.1002/14651858.CD011719.pub3.
31. McCafferty K, Forbes S, Thiemermann C, Yaqoob MM. The challenge of translating ischemic conditioning from animal models to humans: the role of comorbidities. Dis Model Mech. 2014;7(12):1321–33. https://doi.org/10.1242/dmm.016741.
32. Veighey K, Nicholas J, Clayton T, Knight R, Robertson S, Dalton N, et al. Early remote ischaemic preconditioning leads to sustained improvement in allograft function after live donor kidney transplantation: long-term outcomes in the renal protection against ischaemia-reperfusion in transplantation (REPAIR) randomised trial. Br J Anaesth. 2019;123(5):584–91. https://doi.org/10.1016/j.bja.2019.07.019.
33. Pearce L, Davidson S, Yellon D. Does remote ischaemic conditioning reduce inflammation? A focus on innate immunity and cytokine response. Basic Res Cardiol. 2021;116(1):12. https://doi.org/10.1007/s00395-021-00852-0.

34. Jones I, Collins J, Hall N, Heinson A. Transcriptomic analysis of the effect of remote ischaemic conditioning in an animal model of necrotising enterocolitis. Sci Rep. 2024;14(1):10783. https://doi.org/10.1101/2023.10.24.563747.
35. Koike Y, Li B, Ganji N, Zhu H, Miyake H, Chen Y, et al. Remote ischemic conditioning counteracts the intestinal damage of necrotizing enterocolitis by improving intestinal microcirculation. Nat Commun. 2020;11(1):4950. https://doi.org/10.1038/s41467-020-18750-9.
36. Jones I, Tao D, Vagdama B, Orford M, Eaton S, Collins J, Hall N. Remote ischaemic preconditioning reduces intestinal ischaemia reperfusion injury in a newborn rat. J Pediatr Surg. 2023;58(7):1389–98. https://doi.org/10.1016/j.jpedsurg.2022.11.014.

Index

Printed by Printforce, the Netherlands